Training With Kettlebells for Strength and Mobility

The content of this book was carefully researched. However, readers should always consult a qualified medical specialist for individual advice before adopting any new exercise program. This book should not be used as an alternative to seeking specialist medical advice.

All information is supplied without liability. Neither the author nor the publisher will be liable for possible disadvantages, injuries, or damages.

Guido Bruscia

TRAINING WITH KETTLEBELLS FOR STRENGTH AND MOBILITY

OVER 25 FUNCTIONAL TRAINING EXERCISES TO BUILD MUSCLE AND STAY LIMBER

The Ultimate Functional Training Series, Volume II

Meyer & Meyer Sport

Original title: *Allenamento Funzionale – Manuale scientifico*,
© Guido Bruscia, 2013 Elika Srl Editrice via Fossalta 3895-47522 Cesena

Translation: AAA Translation, www.aaatranslation.com

British Library Cataloguing in Publication Data
A catalogue record for this book is available from the British Library

Training With Kettlebells for Strength and Mobility
Maidenhead: Meyer & Meyer Sport (UK) Ltd., 2025
ISBN 978-1-78255-283-3

All rights reserved, especially the right to copy and distribute, including the translation rights. No part of this work may be reproduced—including by photocopy, microfilm or any other means—processed, stored electronically, copied or distributed in any form whatsoever without the written permission of the publisher.

© 2025 by Meyer & Meyer Sport (UK) Ltd.
Aachen, Auckland, Beirut, Cairo, Cape Town, Dubai, Hägendorf, Hongkong, Indianapolis,
Manila, New Dehli, Singapore, Sydney, Tehran, Vienna

Member of the World Sport Publishers' Association (WSPA), www.w-s-p-a.org

Printed by Print Consult GmbH, Munich, Germany
Printed in Slovakia

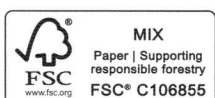

ISBN: 978-1-78255-283-3
E-Mail: info@m-m-sports.com
www.thesportspublisher.com

CONTENTS

ACKNOWLEDGMENTS AND THANKS ... 10

FOREWORD ... 12

INTRODUCTION ... 14

PART I – THEORY ... 16

CHAPTER 1 – THE LOCOMOTOR APPARATUS ... 16

1.1 Presentation ... 17
    1.1.1 The Active Part of the Locomotor Apparatus: Muscles, Tendons, and Ligaments ... 18
    1.1.2 The Passive Part of the Locomotor Apparatus: Bones and Joints ... 19
1.2 Muscle Action ... 21
1.3 Role of the Individual Muscles ... 22
1.4 Articular Features of Muscles ... 23
1.5 Muscular Tissue Features ... 24
1.6 Elements of Biomechanics: Levers ... 25
    1.6.1 Thoughts on Organic Levers ... 28

CHAPTER 2 – ENERGY SYSTEMS ... 29

2.1 Presentation ... 30
2.2 Anaerobic Alactacid System ... 32
2.3 Anaerobic Lactacid System ... 33
2.4 Aerobic System ... 35
2.5 Energy System Interactions ... 37
2.6 VO_2 max and the Anaerobic Threshold ... 38
2.7 Oxygen Debt and EPOC ... 39

CHAPTER 3 – MUSCULAR CONTRACTION 42

3.1	Presentation	43
3.2	Muscular Contraction	45
3.3	Types of Muscle Fibers	46
3.4	Types of Muscular Contraction	48

CHAPTER 4 – TRAINING THEORY 49

4.1	Organic Systems	50
4.2	Training: Presentation	52
4.3	Training Program	54
4.4	Training Theory	55
4.5	Training Parameters	56
4.6	Exercises	58
	4.6.1 Complex exercises	58
	4.6.2 Competition exercises	60

CHAPTER 5 – FUNCTIONAL TRAINING 62

5.1	Kinetic and Kinematic Chains	63
5.2	The Meaning of Functional	64
5.3	The Action-Function Principle	65
5.4	Pebbles Into a Pond	66
5.5	Objectives	68
	5.5.1 What are the Benefits of Functional Training?	68
5.6	Motivations	70
5.7	Functional Training and Pre-athleticism	71
5.8	Functional Training: Other Factors to Develop	72

5.8.1	Training Recruitment	72
	5.8.1.1 Training Recruitment in Adults	73
5.8.2	Strengthening Pivot Muscles	74
5.8.3	Reinforcing the Weak Links in the Kinematic Chains	75
5.8.4	Breaking the Pattern	75

CHAPTER 6 – HIP EXTENSOR CHAIN — 77

6.1	Presentation	78
6.2	Action and Function of the Lower Body	80
6.3	Articular Reality: Long-limbed and Short-limbed Subjects	82
	6.3.1 Consequences	83
6.4	Back Ache, the Iliopsoas, and Evolution	85

CHAPTER 7 – ABDOMINAL FASCIA — 87

7.1	Presentation	88
7.2	Core	90
7.3	Pelvic Floor	90
7.4	Action of the Abdominal Fascia	91
7.5	Function of the Abdominal Fascia	93
7.6	The Centrifuge Principle	95

CHAPTER 8 – SCAPULOHUMERAL GIRDLE — 96

8.1	Presentation	97
8.2	Action of the Scapulohumeral Girdle	98
8.3	Function of the Scapulohumeral Girdle	101
8.4	Grip Types	102

CHAPTER 9 – TIBIAL-TARSAL JOINT AND FOOT 104

9.1 Presentation 105
9.2 Walking 106
9.3 Running 107
9.4 Foot Movements 108

PART II – PRACTICE 109

CHAPTER 10 – KETTLEBELL EXERCISES 109

10.1 Presentation 110
    10.1.1 Origins 110
    10.1.2 Introduction 111
10.2 Lower-body Exercises 112
10.3 Core Training 134
10.4 Upper-body Exercises 142

PART III – OBJECTIVES, METHODS, AND TRAINING PROGRAMS 162

CHAPTER 11 – STRENGTH 162

11.1 The Functional Choice 163
11.2 Strength Training 164
11.3 Strength-training Programs 165

CONTENTS

CHAPTER 12 – HYPERTROPHY 168

12.1 Hypertrophy Training 169
12.2 Cosmetic and Functional Hypertrophy 171
12.3 Functional Hypertrophy-training Programs 172

CHAPTER 13 – SLIMMING 175

13.1 Slimming Training 176
13.2 Lipolytic Paths 177
13.3 Circuit Training 178
    13.3.1 Circuit Training 178
    13.3.2 Cardio-fit Training 181
    13.3.3 Peripheral Heart Action (PHA) Training 185
    13.3.4 Blitz Circuits 188
    13.3.5 Timed Circuits 191
    13.3.6 Boot Camps 193

ETHICS AND CONCLUSIONS 196

ACKNOWLEDGMENTS...

To my family, for never failing to embrace me.

To Ester, my partner and "muse", for our life together.

To my grandmother Sara, 106 years old, still functional today.

To Ernesto Rossi and Sabrina Parrello (and their children Ettore and Giovanni), for their great, true and unconditional friendship.

...AND THANKS

This book was born many years ago and is the work of the author and of all those who have been for him, even if unaware of it, a source of inspiration and ideas:

Emilio They (a friend and master never mourned enough), Marco Neri, Steve Cotter, Michael Boyle, Robert Dos Remedios, Alwin Cosgrove, Martin Rooney, Stuart McGill, Todd Durkin, Josh Henkin, Michol Dalcourt, Gray Cook, Marc Lebert, and many others who, for reasons of space (and memory!), I cannot mention.

Thank you also to all the friends, students, and colleagues who follow me with affection and respect.

ACKNOWLEDGMENTS

Here, too, I can do justice to only a few of them:

Eda Maistrelli, Roberto Braghiroli, Claudio Arena, Emanuele Gollinucci, Roberto Cappelletti, my students at the Hamazon courses in Piombino and Castiglione della Pescaia, Bruno and Serena and the Mensana gym staff in Grosseto, Marco Giannoni and the Palestra Azzurra gym staff in Follonica, Mirko, and Cesare and the Living Club gym staff in Piombino.

Thanks also to the companies that help me with my work:

Elika Editrice

FitnessBest Innovation

Libertas

Ledraplastic

Tecnocomponent

Technogym

Newvitality

Superdry

Xconcept

Vibram Fivefingers

Vistawell

FOREWORD

Ever since humankind appeared on earth, people have always interacted with the environment in their own way.

Civilization has brought infinite advantages to the life of human beings but has also made them weaker and more imperceptive. The senses of smell, hearing and touch, proprioception, and the various organic capacities have all undergone modifications in the course of evolution from our ancestors to the present day. The result is that, while on the one hand we live in heated homes, on the other, a gust of wind is enough to send us to bed with a fever (Marlo Morgan, *E venne chiamata due cuori*).

Galen, one of the fathers of medicine (131-201 AD), wrote in his work *De sanitate tuenda*:

"...This is what I consider as physical exercise or gymnastics, a term connected with the gymnasium, where people go to anoint themselves, enjoy a massage, engage in wrestling, discus throwing or other sporting activities."

More than one thousand years after that, Mercurial recommended discus throwing, rope climbing, race walking, mountain climbing, and long jump as the activities that had the most benefits. People used to train with more or less rudimentary weights: medicine balls, dumbbells, rocks, the trapeze, ropes and still rings.

An athlete had to be strong, fast, and resilient.

FOREWORD

Today, the immense popularity of gyms has produced centers which are extremely well-equipped, sophisticated, and multifunctional. Often, fitness centers imitate outdoor activities with much theatrical effect; they have free-climbing walls meant to resemble jagged, rocky cliffs, water courses and machines that mimic walking, running, and cycling outdoors. And yet, from many quarters, we see signs of a trend in the opposite direction: woodland programs, treetop walks in the woods, life-trails in parks, and a return to body-weight exercises, in which the body is the main training tool. The growing popularity of functional training is a sign that something is changing.

Worn down by the stress of urban life, people are returning to their origins; they are feeling the need for a stroll, a run, a different kind of muscular workout unconstrained by machines or showy equipment. They are looking for woods or meadows.

Nature all around, and, overhead, the sky as the only limit.

INTRODUCTION

When we talk about education, we refer to a system of knowledge which involves different fields of learning and is constantly evolving.

Gym activity requires the knowledge of physiology, anatomy, and biomechanics. Knowledge of nutrition and supplements also has proven to have an influence on sports performance and on results, and not just in terms of achievements. Also, in recent years, several studies have overturned many ideas and misconceptions connected with the world of sports.

Knowledge is an imperfect journey, full of trial and error. To these facts we have to add, of course, exercise practice, an empirical science which is by no means a given. Contrary to most beliefs, practice does not make us perfect: It is perfect practice that makes us perfect. The objective of education is to create professionalism, a word which, today like never before, plays a fundamental role in a coach's assessment. A professional is someone who provides a unique performance. Let's not forget this.

INTRODUCTION

WARNING

This textbook has been written with the average fitness enthusiast in mind.

For this reason, I have glossed over issues which aren't strictly germane to the theme and sacrificed the purely technical definition of several concepts in favor of a more direct, straightforward language.

Medicalese doesn't help in assimilating concepts.

RESOLUTIONS

In 2004, at a personal trainers convention, I lectured on:

"Functional training for the lower limbs: A new perspective." In subsequent years, I studied the functional subject in depth, comparing my findings with those of several gurus in the USA, Spain, Switzerland, Germany, Slovenia, and Italy.

Functional training changes your life. Not your sporting life, which is focused on the search for optimal performance or, accordingly, for hypertrophy and super-toned bodies. Functional training simply makes people feel better, making them more active, stronger, tougher. In a few weeks, you will notice that your health is changing and that your physical efficiency and the well-being you are enjoying today have reached new heights. All this is the result of an optimization of factors which contribute to building a new body. It will not just be a matter of being more toned; there will be the awareness of feeling efficient for the first time.

Your body is like a custom-made outfit: It is the best place to live in.

All you have to do is try.

PART I – THEORY

CHAPTER 1

THE LOCOMOTOR APPARATUS

1.1 PRESENTATION

Every time we think about a sporting activity, we associate it with the concept of *motion*.

This process is so widespread and natural that we don't think about its underlying reason *why*. During courses, students who are interested in and passionate about training sometimes ask me why it is necessary to know stuff that has no apparent connection with a horizontal bench or a squat.

The answer is that gymnastics, in its broadest sense, is an empirical science; it stands apart from scientific bases which interact constantly with sporting exercise in gyms or outdoors. For this reason, you will often find not only various definitions, but also examples which refer back to practice.

The locomotor apparatus is the structure that allows a person to move in relation to space and the outside world. For practical purposes, it is subdivided into an active part and a passive part. The active part is made up of muscles, tendons, and ligaments. The inactive part is composed of bones and joints. Each is briefly discussed in the following sections.

1.1.1 The active part of the locomotor apparatus: Muscles, tendons, and ligaments

MUSCLES

The term *muscle*, from the Latin *musculus* (from *mus*, rat, because some movements are reminiscent of a rat darting about), indicates an organ made of biological tissue with the ability to contract.

The muscles are subdivided into:

- Smooth, or involuntary, muscles
  Commanded by the autonomic nervous system, they encase the walls of several organs and corporeal systems, enabling or improving their functionality with their contraction.

- Striated skeletal, or voluntary, muscles
  Commanded by the central nervous system, they encase the skeleton, and, by their contraction (shortening), they determine the bone levers' movement.

A peculiar type of striated muscle is the myocardium, which is commanded by the autonomic nervous system.

TENDONS

Tendons are bands of connective tissue with poor elasticity, and their function is to anchor the muscles to the bones. Their role is to transmit tension from muscles to the bone levers, thus allowing their movement.

THE LOCOMOTOR APPARATUS

LIGAMENTS

Ligaments are sheaves of connective tissue with varying percentages of collagen fibers that link bones at the joints. The ligaments' purpose is to limit articular movement which would risk creating lesions were it to continue. For example, the knee's collateral medial and lateral ligaments support the anterior and posterior cruciate ligaments in limiting the articulation's intra- and extrarotation movements in order to avoid lesions to the knee itself.

1.1.2 The passive part of the locomotor apparatus: Bones and joints

BONES

Bones are specialized tissues with great mechanical resistance. They are divided into:

- Long bones (humerus, femur, tibia, radius): These are composed of an elongated body known as *diaphysis* and by terminal extremities known as *epiphysis*; they determine raw movements, which are characterized by wide articular excursions.
- Short bones (vertebrae): They have a similar diameter in all three spatial dimensions.
- Irregular bones (facial bones, the patella): These bones are characterized by variable dimensions and shape.
- Flat bones (pelvis, sternum, skull): Their function is protecting internal organs.

Don't be misled by bone tissue in the passive part of the locomotor apparatus: The bone is a highly active and dynamic tissue. In fact, from birth, the bone undergoes a remodeling process, involving the change and overlap of catabolic and anabolic phases. The catabolic phases are stimulated by micro organelles called *osteoclasts*, and the anabolic phases are activated by other specialized cells called *osteoblasts*. The piezoelectric effect gives the input for an increased bone tissue synthesis activity.

What does it involve? During motor activity, bone segment compression generates an electric depolarization of the bone membrane at the load points. This creates a greater localized need for the reconstructive osteoblasts. This explains why weight training, as demonstrated by several studies, has turned out to be an excellent remedy to contrast osteoporosis.

JOINTS

Joints are the junction hubs between two or more bone segments around which bones rotate.

According to their configuration and degree of mobility, joints can be classified as follows:

- **Synarthroses:** These are fixed, fibrous joints with little or no possibility of movement.
- **Amphiarthroses:** These joints are semi-mobile; they are often cartilaginous (e.g., vertebrae).
- **Diarthroses:** These are the mobile, synovial joints capable of a greater degree of movement. In terms of movement range, the most significant are the enarthroses (e.g., shoulder and hip), with spherical-shaped, multi-axial articular surfaces.

1.2 MUSCLE ACTION

For clarity, I have simplified the different muscular actions, adding the technical definition in parentheses.

- **Flexion:** When two bone segments move closer to each other (the moving part draws away from the horizontal plane). Example: brachial biceps, femoral biceps
- **Extension:** When two bone segments move away from each other (the moving part draws nearer to the horizontal plane). Example: brachial triceps, femoral quadriceps
- **Adduction:** When a bone segment draws closer to the median sagittal line (the moving part draws closer to the sagittal plane). Example: thigh adductors group
- **Abduction:** When a bone segment draws away from the median sagittal line (the moving plane draws away from the median sagittal plane). Examples: gluteus minimus and gluteus medius, high tensor fascia, deltoid
- **Torsion:** Movement of the trunk around the vertical axis.
- **Rotation:** Movement of a limb on its longitudinal axis.
- **Intrarotation:** Rotation of a bone segment in the medial direction, in other words, toward the inside (movement toward the anterior frontal plane).
- **Extrarotation:** Rotation of a bone segment in the lateral direction, in other words, toward the outside (movement toward the posterior frontal plane).

Each muscle performs several movements, which must be differentiated in order to better define exercises and their completion. For example, flexion and extension take place when the limbs aren't bearing weight. Bending, however, takes place when the limbs are bearing weight, as when completing a push-up. We may therefore notice that what is commonly referred to as flexing the arms is defined more correctly as bending the arms.

1.3 ROLE OF THE INDIVIDUAL MUSCLES

Based on the role they play in movement, we may differentiate muscles as:

- **Agonist muscles:** They play the main role in a specific action. Example: pectoral muscles in the horizontal bench press.
- **Antagonist muscles:** In the same action, they play an opposite role to the agonist muscles. Example: the trapezius muscle in the horizontal bench press.
- **Synergistic muscles** (from the Greek *sun-ergo*, "working together"): They help and support the agonist muscles. Examples: the triceps and anterior deltoid muscles in the horizontal bench press.
- **Neutralizing muscles** (stabilizers): They stabilize a bone segment, allowing other muscles to execute a certain action.
- **Fixator muscles:** They act as stabilizers, but they that is not their only role. They block a segment in the position that is appropriate to a movement or an action. Examples: pectoralis and latissimus dorsi muscles in parallel bars exercises.

1.4 ARTICULAR FEATURES OF MUSCLES

In gyms, muscle articulation is mostly disregarded, if not completely ignored.

Yet muscle articulation is of fundamental importance in understanding how to teach various exercise methods. Muscle articulation is defined as:

- **monoarticular,** those muscles that control only one joint and are inserted on bone levers that are paired by one joint only; and
- **bi- or multiarticular,** those muscles that cross over two or more joints.

In order to understand the importance of this distinction, let me remind you that when a muscle is biarticular, it should be stimulated with biarticular movements in order to be fully trained.

The most common example is that of the biceps brachii. Though it is a biarticular muscle, the biceps brachii is usually trained with monoarticular movements—the upper arm is kept steady against the trunk while only the forearm moves. To be clear, the monoarticular movement in this case isn't wrong, but it is nevertheless incomplete.

1.5 MUSCULAR TISSUE FEATURES

The features of muscular tissue are the following:

- **Contractility:** a muscle's ability to shorten.
- **Extensibility:** a muscle's ability to lengthen.
- **Elasticity:** the muscle tissue's ability to return to the initial length from a stretching position (the time factor needs to be evaluated, too).
- **Tonicity:** a very low-intensity electrical message which is always present within the muscle, even when at rest.

A common mistake is assuming that stretching helps only to elongate the muscle. In reality, there are many more effects of stretching:

- Extensibility
- Elasticity
- Articular flexibility
- Elongation of the connective tissue

For many years now, the concept of analytic stretching, in other words, stretching a single muscle or articular segment, has been surpassed in favor of systemic stretching, which involves longer muscular and articular chains.

More accurately, today we talk about mobilization, with reference to

- the joints, where muscles connect; and
- the connective tissue which covers the muscles and is less extensible than the joints; this means that when you talk about stretching a muscle, actually the range of the stretch is deeply influenced by the elasticity of the tissue that covers it.

THE LOCOMOTOR APPARATUS

1.6 ELEMENTS OF BIOMECHANICS: LEVERS

Biomechanics is the science that studies the law of mechanical actions in living systems.

Sports biomechanics studies a human being's movement within the process of physical exercise.

The study of biomechanics is essential when approaching any motor or sporting activity in order to identify

- the body's structure and motor functions; and
- the specific technique of the sport being studied.

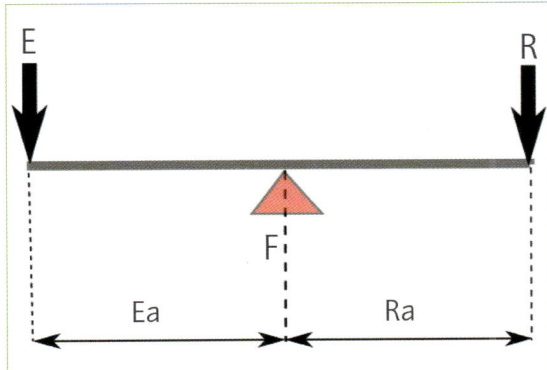

Lever in balance

A *lever* is a simple machine consisting of a rigid segment tied to a fixed point called a fulcrum (F), upon which two forces of equal strength but opposite direction are applied, called effort (E) and resistance (R).

The distance from the fulcrum to the point where resistance is applied is called the resistance arm (Ra); the distance from the fulcrum to the point where effort is applied is called the effort arm (Ea).

A lever is in balance when the resistance and effort arms are equal.

A lever is disadvantageous when the resistance arm is greater than the effort arm.

A lever is advantageous when the effort arm is greater than the resistance arm.

If we think about it, we realize that our skeletal system is a set of levers:

- Bones are the rigid segments.
- The fulcrum consists of the various joints that are involved.
- Resistance consists of the weight (load) we apply to the various levers.
- Effort consists of the muscles which contrast the weight's action.

The application point of resistance (i.e., where the resistance arm departs from) is the point of contact between the weight and the locomotor apparatus. The application point of effort (i.e., where the effort arm departs from) is where the muscle inserts into the bone segment. There are three types of levers in the human body, separated according to the distribution of the effort and resistance forces and the fulcrum around which the various bone segments hinge:

Type 1: Inter-fulcrum lever

The fulcrum is always positioned between effort and resistance. As we saw, a lever is advantageous, disadvantageous, or in balance according to whether the effort arm is greater than, smaller than, or equal to the resistance arm.

Example: a pair of scissors, a 45-degree calf exercise at the press machine.

THE LOCOMOTOR APPARATUS

Type 2: Inter-resistance lever

From its name we can deduce that resistance will always be positioned between the fulcrum and effort. The effort arm, therefore, is always greater than the resistance arm. The lever is always advantageous.

Example: nutcracker, standing calf raise exercise.

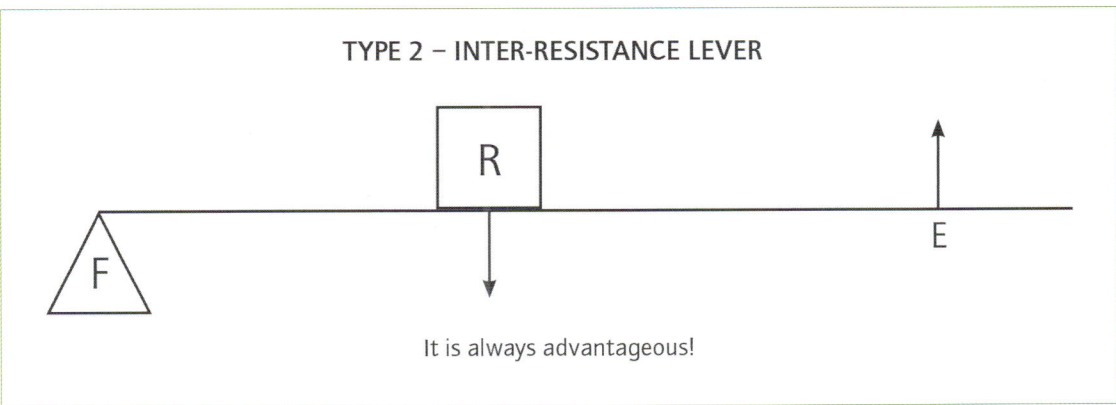

Type 3: Inter-effort lever

The same logic applies: Effort will always be located between fulcrum and resistance. The resistance arm is always greater than the effort arm. The lever is disadvantageous.

Example: tweezers, biceps.

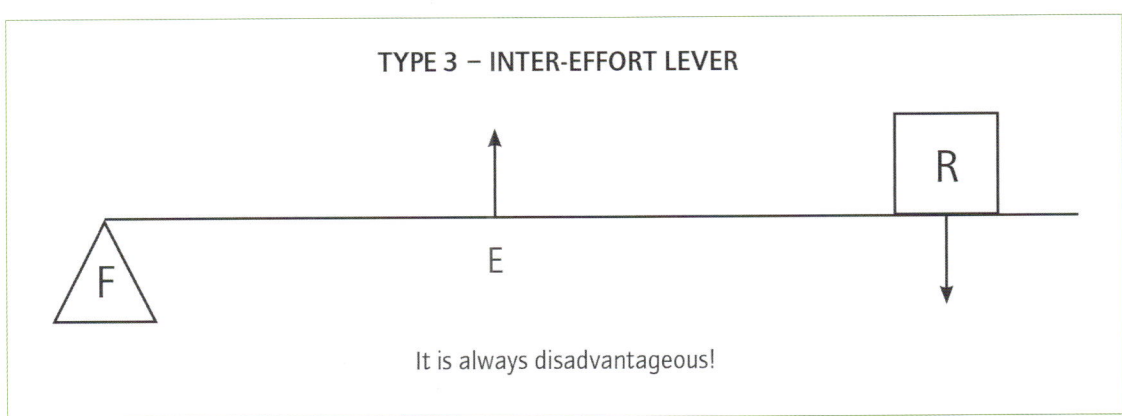

1.6.1 Thoughts on organic levers

The majority of organic levers, at least when it comes to long bones (i.e., great locomotion), are type 3. Our body has opted for a predominance of disadvantageous levers. Why? Because this type of lever, though disadvantageous in terms of strength, allows wider movements and greater articular excursions and at high speeds. In practical terms, the evolutionary choice has been toward greater speed. (Let's keep these features in mind.

CHAPTER 2

2.1 PRESENTATION

Life on Earth has evolved along the energy road, consuming energy economically and obtaining it easily. All living organisms now extinct (not because of human intervention) were inefficient energy systems and, as such, extremely wasteful. Living, making the body function, or performing any action requires energy. We can define *energy* as the ability to carry out a task. Specifically, a muscle is a chemodynamic machine; in other words, it functions through chemical reactions.

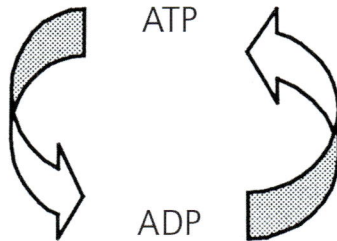

In order to convey a concept, it is useful to use imagery, visualizing the concept in pictures. To simplify the following chemical reaction, I will use imagery. Imagine a car. The model is called Man. Its fuel is adenosine triphosphate, or simply ATP. The human machine's universal fuel (its gasoline) is a molecule possessed of a high degree of chemical energy.

ENERGY SYSTEMS

Our cells burn ATP continuously, and they are always synthesizing new ATP to obtain a supply of energy.

The gasoline's combustion in the car, Man, comes from the following reaction:

$$ATP \rightarrow ATPase \rightarrow ADP + P + Energy$$
$$Energy = (7.3\ kcal/mole)$$

ATP breaks down into adenosine diphosphate, and this reaction produces energy.

The adenosine triphosphatase enzyme catalyzes the reaction (enzymes are substances which catalyze—they influence the speed of biochemical reactions, increasing or decreasing).

The amount of ATP present within cells allows them to work for a few seconds only. So how do they continue to work over time? They activate makeshift energy systems, with the objective of producing ATP (energy) according to the intensity and duration of the activity required. Intensity and duration cannot go hand in hand; they are two inversely proportional parameters. The more intensity (i.e., energy supply) required during an activity, the shorter the activity will be. Conversely, a lower intensity will allow a longer workout. Think about sprinting: You can run 100 m [109 yd] very fast, but you can't keep up the same speed to run, for example, 3,000 m [3,280 yd].

2.2 ANAEROBIC ALACTACID (CREATINE PHOSPHATE) SYSTEM

Let's imagine:

Car: Man
Model: Formula 1
Fuel: ATP + CP

This system is used when an immediate supply of energy is needed for a very high-intensity but short-duration workout: 0-20 min (optimized at around 13 min).

What does the name tell us?

Anaerobic means there is no presence of oxygen; *alactacid* means that no lactic acid is produced.

We use a process called *phosphorylation:* The energy level of a substance is increased by binding it to a phosphoric group.

How is the energy supplied? Let's review the basic reaction:

$$ATP \rightarrow ATPase \rightarrow ADP + P + Energy$$

In this reaction, ATP breaks down into ADP. At this stage, ATP gets recharged by creatine phosphate (CP). CP doesn't supply energy directly, but it supports ADP, retransforming it into ATP, allowing the reaction to continue.

$$ADP + CP \rightarrow cpkase \rightarrow C + ATP$$
(Loehmann's mono-enzyme reaction)

The concentration of CP in the muscle is four to six times higher compared to that of ATP; this allows the energy supply to last a little longer compared to using ATP only.

Examples of sporting activities requiring CP for energy: 60-100 m [65.6-109 yd] sprint, long jump, high jump, strength training

2.3 ANAEROBIC LACTACID SYSTEM

Let's imagine:

Car: Man
Model: Turbo-diesel sedan
Fuel: Glycogen/ATP

This system is used in performances that require a high energy supply for a medium-short duration. Let's analyze the name again. *Anaerobic* means in the absence of oxygen; *lactacid* means that there is lactic acid, or lactate, production. The ATP molecules are stored inside the muscles and the liver in the form of a complex sugar, an animal polysaccharide: glycogen (you can imagine diesel fuel). ATP is produced when glycogen breaks down into glucose, producing pyruvic acid and, subsequently, lactic acid.

This energy supply process is fast; it allows a high- to medium-intensity workout between 20 sec and 2 min (optimized around 30-40 sec).

The longer time required for the supply of energy compared to the anaerobic alactacid system is due to the 10 chemical reactions that lead to the breakdown of the molecules mentioned above.

Energy comes from the muscular glycogen and the hepatic glucose, according to the following steps:

$$\text{GLUCOSE} \\ \downarrow \\ \text{2 ATP} \\ \downarrow \\ \text{PYRUVIC ACID} \\ \downarrow \\ \text{LACTIC ACID}$$

When one glucose molecule breaks down into pyruvic acid, two ATP molecules are formed.

This process is also known as *anaerobic glycolysis*.

This being a high-intensity activity with low utilization of oxygen, a highly acidic environment forms inside the muscles. Pyruvic acid binds to two excess H+ ions, producing lactic acid.

$$ADP + P + glucose \rightarrow ATP + lactic\ acid$$

When the lactate build-up becomes excessively high, the muscle's contractile capacity is inhibited (hypoxia).

What is the fate of lactic acid? Once the exercise is finished, it is partly used as fuel but it is chiefly re-converted into pyruvic acid and re-stocked in the muscles as muscular and hepatic glycogen (Cori's cycle).

Lactic acid isn't the cause for post-training pains!

ENERGY SYSTEMS

2.4 AEROBIC SYSTEM (AEROBIC GLYCOLYSIS OR OXIDATIVE PHOSPHORYLATION IN MITOCHONDRIA)

Let's imagine:

Car: Man
Model: MPV car
Fuel: Macronutrients/ATP

This system is used for all activities ranging from very low to medium intensity, lasting from a few minutes to some hours. Let's take a closer look.

Aerobic means the presence of oxygen is required.

Beyond the 2-min mark, only the presence of oxygen still allows glucose transformation; if the activity lasts longer than this, the system begins to activate processes which use stored fat as fuel. Compared to carbohydrates, lipids have a more unfavorable ratio between hydrogen and oxygen, and this explains the need to capture oxygen from outside to metabolize them. Proteins, too, provide energy within this system but in a lower percentage (3-5%).The process, also called *oxidative phosphorylation*, takes place within mitochondria, the cell's miniature power stations. The start is similar to the anaerobic lactacid system:

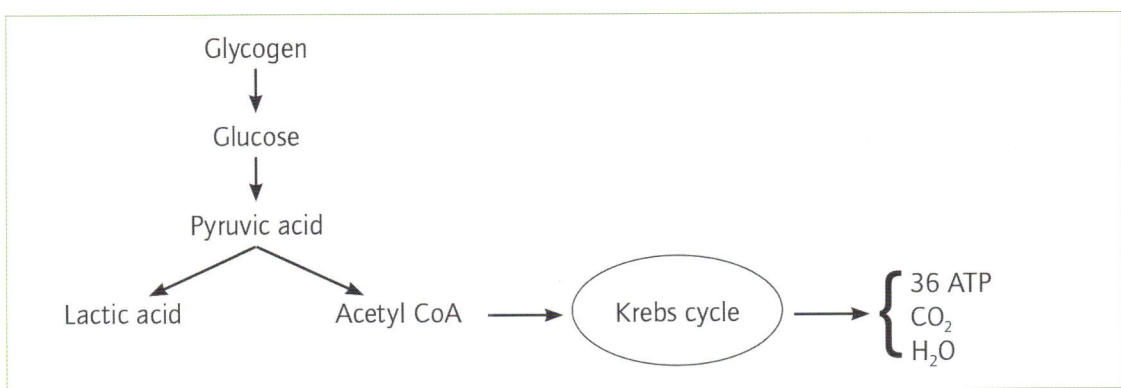

Because this is a reduced-intensity activity, pyruvic acid is transformed into acetyl-coenzyme A and transferred to the mitochondria, entering the Krebs cycle. The latter is like a metabolic furnace inside which the glucose molecule is completely broken down, generating 36 ATP, carbon dioxide, and water molecules.

In order to produce ATP, the aerobic system needs hydrogen. This is supplied by the Krebs cycle, exploiting oxidation (i.e., the removal of hydrogen) of food-derived compounds. Hydrogen is then transported to the respiratory chain via NAD (nicotinamide-nucleotide) and FAD (flavin adenine dinucleotide) up to the final receptor, oxygen, generating water.

Summarizing, the aerobic system is the result of two events:

1. Substrata breakdown, with production of hydrogen and carbon dioxide (Krebs cycle).
2. Hydrogen transportation to the respiratory chain, forming water.

2.5 ENERGY SYSTEM INTERACTIONS

It is important to understand how the three energy systems cooperate.

The basic mechanism used by our body is the aerobic system. All the activities in our normal daily life take place at a low intensity and do not require a high amount of energy. This means that the aerobic system can comfortably provide the energy for all our daily activities. Whenever more intense efforts beyond the aerobic system's capacity are needed, the anaerobic systems work together with the aerobic system.

Note that in supplying energy, the three energy systems do not alternate like a relay. So when the synthesized ATP is active, it does not pass the baton to the anaerobic alactacid system, which in turn does not pass it to the anaerobic lactacid one. Instead, the three systems work together in parallel but also in different percentages, according to the type of effort, its duration, and the related demand for energy.

2.6 VO$_2$MAX AND THE ANAEROBIC THRESHOLD

The concepts connected to the terms *VO$_2$max, anaerobic threshold,* and *oxygen debt* are important.

VO$_2$max, or maximum aerobic power, is in practical terms the organism's maximum capacity for synthesizing ATP using aerobics exclusively. It has actually been observed that this figure is more the result of a theoretical calculation than something reproducible in a lab or, even harder, in real life. An athlete is capable of maintaining an effort equal to VO$_2$max for no more than 10 min. Why? Besides a long list of factors—the majority of them genetic—the fact remains that at the experimental level it has been observed that well before reaching this limit the body begins to produce lactic acid. For this reason, at least in fitness training, the concept of anaerobic threshold has become increasingly important.

The **anaerobic threshold** is the maximum level of physical effort the organism can sustain without accumulating lactate in the blood. Above that heart rate the organism begins accumulating lactic acid because it cannot dispose of it as fast as it can produce it. The outcome is the fast onset of fatigue.

ENERGY SYSTEMS

2.7 OXYGEN DEBT AND EPOC

Oxygen debt is the increased uptake of oxygen needed to remove excess lactic acid that is created by the increased synthesis of ATP which results from anaerobic physical exercise. What does this mean? We have seen that when you start a motor activity, there is an increase in the body's energy requirements. At the outset, the aerobic system isn't immediately available unless the activity is at a very low intensity.

The body, therefore, requires help from the anaerobic systems, increasing the oxygen debt. The greater the intensity of the activity, the larger the debt. As soon as the effort is over, the body pays its debt by increasing oxygen uptake from the outside in order to restore phosphates and remove the lactic acid produced.

Dash or sprint for 20-30 sec. Now stop. What are you doing? You're panting. Your trunk leans forward, and your hands are on your knees. In order to increase your thoracic cavity's capacity, you inhale as much oxygen as possible from the air around you. This is the increased oxygen uptake.

Any exercise which involves the development of power above VO_2max is defined as *supramaximal*.

An oxygen debt can also be incurred as a result of a supramaximal load imposed on muscles; the oxidative machine intervenes in this case, too, at the end of the performance. However, in the ensuing recovery phase, the oxygen uptake exceeds the volume of the deficit. It's as though you're paying your debt with interest.

Margaria[1], R. (1938) has shown how the O_2 consumption curve during recovery can be split into four components:

1. **Constant component:** it depends on the subject's metabolism at rest.
2. **Fast component:** payment of the debt's alactacid fraction at a decreasing rate; lactate halves every 30 sec.
3. **Slow component:** payment of the lactacid debt at a slowly decreasing rate because of the energy cost of the renewed glycogen synthesis originating from lactic acid.
4. **Slow, long-lasting component:** attributed to the stimulus effect of the exercise on the metabolism at rest.

---

[1] Margaria R. (1938). Sulla fisiologia e specialmente sul consumo energetico della marcia e della corsa a varia velocità ed inclinazione del terreno, in *Atti Accademia Nazionale dei Lincei* 7, 299-368.

ENERGY SYSTEMS

With regards to this, studies show how the more intense a training session is, the higher the metabolism remains for a longer period of time in order to compensate the oxygen debt.

Recently, the concept of oxygen debt has been included in the wider concept of EPOC (excess post-exercise oxygen consumption). EPOC includes not just the oxygen debt but also the domino-effect adaptations which depend on it:

- Payment of the alactacid debt.
- Payment of the lactacid debt.
- Increased body temperature.
- Thermogenic effect caused by catecholamines.
- Renewed lactate synthesis.
- Renewed phosphagen synthesis.
- Lactate and blood oxygenation.
- High cardiac frequency.

CHAPTER 3

3.1 PRESENTATION

We have seen in the preceding chapters a presentation of the locomotor apparatus and of the energy systems through which the body acquires energy for movement.

Let's now focus our attention on the muscles, specifically on the processes which lead to muscular contraction and on the phenomena that result.

Let's introduce the main players:

1. The central nervous system (CNS). It consists of the brain, the cerebellum, and the spinal cord. From here voluntary muscular contraction originates through a nerve impulse.
2. The drive units. They consist of a body called *motor neuron*, an electric cable, the axon (including an insulating substance, the myelin sheath), and the muscular fibers stemming from it. The drive units' task is to carry the nerve impulse from the CNS to the muscle. The movement input reaches the muscle from the drive unit via a neurotransmitter (i.e., a substance which transmits a nerve impulse, called acetylcholine [Ach]).

TRAINING WITH KETTLEBELLS FOR STRENGTH AND MOBILITY

3. The muscles. Each muscle is composed of a muscle belly surrounded by a sheath of connective tissue called *epimysium*.

- *Muscular fibers.* Inside the muscle there are groups of fibers bundled together in primary sheaths, or fascicles, encased by the perimysium. The primary sheaths are formed by muscular fibers encased by the epimysium; muscular fibers are in turn made of myofibrils, sheathed by the endomysium.

3.2 MUSCULAR CONTRACTION

Viewed through an electron microscope, myofibrils appear as long filaments divided up into compartments by darker strips. Myofibrils can be compared with a train. The single cars, segmented by the Z lines, are called sarcomeres, and they constitute the cell's essential contractile unit. Inside each car (sarcomere) are two main regulatory proteins that partial overlap: actin (which is thinner) and myosin (larger, shaped like an oar or a golf club). We also find two other regulatory proteins, troponin and tropomyosin, interposed between the actin and myosin.

Skeletal muscle structure.

Actin and myosin.

Voluntary muscular contraction originates from the brain, goes through the cerebellum (movement is intermediary, making it fluid and coordinated), and reaches the spinal cord. From the spinal cord, the drive units incite the release of calcium ions from small cisterns called T-shaped tubules by releasing acetylcholine. The calcium ions bind with tropomyosin and troponin, canceling their inhibiting effect on actin and myosin. At this stage, the two main regulatory proteins come into contact. In the presence of ATP, the myosin heads attach to actin, pulling it and making it slide above them.

This sliding process is applied to every sarcomere inside the muscle and leads to its shortening or contraction (Huxley's myofilament sliding theory).

3.3 TYPES OF MUSCLE FIBERS

There exist two main types of muscular fibers, both possessing very different chemical and physical features.

- **Type I fibers,** or red fibers, or slow-twitch fibers.
  They are small and rich in mitochondria. They produce small tensions but are endowed with significant endurance.

- **Type II fibers,** or white fibers, or fast-twitch fibers.
  They are larger and produce high tensions but only for a short time. They hypertrophy very easily and are divided in two subgroups: type IIx and type IIa.

1. *Type IIx fibers* are known as pure white fibers and also as fast glycotic, with very few mitochondria, high tensile capacity and very limited endurance.
2. *Type IIa fibers,* or fast oxidative glycotic are also called intermediate fibers, since they share both some of the red and white fibers' characteristics: a good percentage of mitochondria, fine tensile capacity, and moderate endurance.

The percentage of fibers which innervate a specific muscle points to the type of training needed for it as well. For example, if hypertrophy is the objective, a muscle with a high percentage of white fibers will need to be trained with high weight loads, few repetitions, maximal or submaximal tensions, and long recovery periods. However, a muscle with a high percentage of red fibers will need to be trained with lighter weight loads, medium to high repetitions, and markedly submaximal tensions, though continuous and isotensive.

For this reason, the table indicating the statistical percentages of the various muscle fibers found within a muscle can provide excellent indications for a training program.

MUSCULAR CONTRACTION

Table of the percentage of various fibers in some muscles.

Muscle	% STa*	% FTa*	% FTb*
Adductor brevis	45	15	40
Brachial biceps	50	-	50
Femoral biceps	65	10	25
Deltoid	60	-	40
Gastrocnemius	50	20	30
Gracilis	55	15	30
Adductor magnus	55	15	30
Latissimus dorsi	50	-	50
Gluteus maximus	50	20	30
Pectoralis major	42	-	58
Iliopsoas	50	-	50
Psoas	50	20	30
Rectus abdominis	46	-	54
Rectus femoris	45	15	40
Rhomboid	45	-	55
Semimembranosus	50	15	35
Soleus	75	15	10
Tensor fascia lata	70	10	20
Tibialis anterior	70	10	20
Trapezius	54	-	64
Brachial triceps	33	-	67
Vastus intermedius	50	15	35
Vastus lateralis	45	20	35
Vastus medialis	50	15	35

* STa = Slow-twitch fibres
 FTA = Fast-twitch fibres
 FTB = Fast-twitch fibres

3.4 TYPES OF MUSCULAR CONTRACTION

Muscular contraction is defined as the physiological means through which muscular fibers are recruited once the nerve impulse has arrived and given a sufficient amount of energy. Muscular contractions divide into two groups: static contractions and dynamic contractions. In static contractions the muscle doesn't modify its length, even though tension is developed. Dynamic contractions determine, on the other hand, a modification in the muscle's length.

1. **Static (isometric) contractions.** The muscle develops an amount of tension equal to the resistance applied, doesn't modify its length (the distance between muscular insertions is unchanged), and doesn't generate any output (in the physical sense, meaning there is no displacement). Isometric contractions may be
   - maximal: tension is applied with an unmovable load; or
   - stationary: the movement is voluntarily interrupted.

2. **Dynamic (non-isometric) contractions.** The muscle develops tension and changes its length, producing an output; the distance between the insertions changes during contraction. Non-isometric contractions may be:
   - concentric (positive): the tension developed is such as to overcome the applied tension; the muscle shortens, and the insertions draw closer.
   - eccentric (negative): the tension developed is less than the resistance applied; the muscle lengthens, the insertions draw farther.
   - Isotonic: the muscle shortens, developing a constant tension for the entire length of the shortening period. Actually, in reality, isotonic contractions do not exist. The tension developed varies as the lever varies. We can simulate isotonic contraction only with machines featuring physiological camshafts.
   - Isokinetic: the muscle generates the maximum amount of tension throughout the movement, shortening at constant speed (specific isokinetic equipment is used).
   - Auxotonic: the tension generated increases progressively as the muscle shortens (e.g., an elastic band).
   - Plyometric: explosive, concentric contractions immediately preceded by eccentric contractions; this exploits the energy accumulated within the muscle's elastic structures.

CHAPTER 4

4.1 ORGANIC SYSTEMS

Our body has 11 systems. Each system is made up of different organs. These 11 systems are responsible for complex physical functions. In other words, each system has a specific goal. The physical functions are:

PROTECTION

1. *Integumentary system:* the skin protects the underlying tissues, regulates body temperature, and synthesizes chemical substances and hormones.

SUPPORT AND MOVEMENT

1. *Skeletal system.*
2. *Muscular system.*

COMMUNICATIONS, CONTROL, AND INTEGRATION

1. *Nervous system:* it takes care of the generation, transmission, integration, and gathering of specialized nerve impulses.
2. *Endocrine system:* hormones are the main regulators of our metabolism, growth, development, reproduction, and other activities.

TRAINING THEORY

TRANSPORT AND DEFENSE

1. *Cardiovascular system.*
2. *Lymphatic system.*

TRANSFORMATION, REGULATION, AND MAINTENANCE

1. *Respiratory system.*
2. *Digestive system.*
3. *Urinary system:* kidneys cleanse waste from the blood. Inside the kidneys, the waste is transformed in urine.

REPRODUCTION AND GROWTH

1. *Reproductive system:* it guarantees the genetic code's survival.

All these systems exist in a state of equilibrium called homeostasis. The body constantly strives for equilibrium, reacting with negative feedback mechanisms to any sudden change.

Every time there is a sudden rise or fall in any system's parameters, the body activates certain physiological responses in order to bring the parameters back to the preexisting state of equilibrium.

Now, to avoid adopting the superior attitude of "experts" who train a different muscle group every day, you must understand that the stress applied on any system is also reflected on others and forces them to adapt.

Try this: Do a set of squats until you are exhausted. The effects? Respiration is fatigued, so therefore the cardiovascular and cardiorespiratory systems are stressed. The hip extensor chain—gluteus and quadriceps—is fatigued, and this means that the musculoskeletal system has been activated. Thighs and legs feel heavy, indicating the production of, the sign of an increased hormonal response (involving the endocrine system). We know also that among the physiological responses our body activates as a reaction to a stressful stimulus, such as training, there is an immune response. So another system is activated. Do you need to know more?

TRAINING WITH KETTLEBELLS FOR STRENGTH AND MOBILITY

4.2 TRAINING: PRESENTATION

How to define training?

A person decides to start running, jumping, and doing push-ups with the arms and legs, doing this regularly until the onset of fatigue, trying to improve.

This means that this person is adding an extra energy stress (basal metabolism) to the daily energy consumption. This is not enough. This stress doesn't simply translate into greater energy consumption; it also translates into peripheral stress applied to the locomotor apparatus, which alters the equilibrium of the 11 organic systems that regulate this person's body. Sports training in physiology is defined as a stressor (i.e., a stressful stimulus). Compared to normal daily activities, stress is a series of factors that alter organic homeostasis, inducing a systemic response from the body. The systemic response is specific, depending on the type of stress involved, and non-specific, which is typical of all stress situations.

Selye's Law.

TRAINING THEORY

In order to be productive, stress must specifically have continuity (frequency), effort (intensity), and duration (volume). Training frequency determines the essential aspect that generates supercompensatory adaptations: recovery. This is what Selye's Law, or the law of supercompensation, says:

Following a stress situation, the organism activates a series of non-specific and specific responses involving the whole body, leading to a series of consequential adaptations after a suitable recovery.

The body effectively reacts to any stressful stimulus with a response and adaptation that are consequential and proportional to the stimulus received. Supercompensation will take place only after the organism has restored the conditions from before the onset of the training stress.

Improving a specific feature does not take place during the training session but during the following recovery phase; continuously subjecting someone to new training stress without allowing the body full recovery between sessions will cause overtraining syndrome (OTS).

4.3 TRAINING PROGRAM

Let's assume that training is the administration of stress, an additional burden to normal relational life that alters organic homeostasis in order to obtain a consequential response and adaptation (supercompensation).

In figure I (see page 58), the training stimulus is excessively rarefied.

This situation doesn't generate a chronic additional burden for the body, so there is no supercompensating adaptation.

In figure II, training stimuli which are excessively close to one another prevent supercompensating adaptation, quickly leading to overtraining.

In figure III, correctly scheduling training sessions over time leads to improvement.

You will notice in the definition of training the word *administration* is a pharmaceutical or medical term.

It was not chosen randomly. If training is to be scientific, its elaboration and training stimulus must be equally scientific.

Do remember: Each muscular structure has its own specific stimulus. This is a fact, even though it is true that certain stimuli, training for strength and its components, lead to improvement also in other structures, features, and characteristics.

Why? Any response is systemic: It involves the whole body.

Therefore a training program is the schedule of the stress (load) an individual must apply to his or her organic systems in order to obtain physiological modifications and related adaptations.

4.4 TRAINING THEORY

Let's now see which rules must be followed in order for training to yield results over time.

OVERLOAD

In order to induce physiological modifications leading to performance improvement, we must apply a training stimulus that is at least higher than that generated by normal daily life. This implies that once certain adaptations have been obtained, it will be necessary to train with workloads increasing in magnitude (load progressiveness) in order to further improve.

SPECIFICITY

A training stimulus will generate specific modifications in relation to the type of overload applied. Effectively, the benefits obtained from power training and those derived from aerobic training aren't interchangeable. In power training, we will have modifications typical of power training, while in aerobic training, there will be aerobic modifications.

INDIVIDUALITY

Given the multiple, infinite factors which differentiate one person from another, it isn't advisable to apply the same training program to all people, using identical stimuli, loads, and exercises. Training must be programmed according to the person , bearing in mind his or her physical, structural, and metabolic characteristics.

LOSS OF TRAINING

The effects of training are transitory and reversible proportional to the type, intensity, and duration of the applied stimulus. After 10-14 days of rest, there is a regression in several motor components already achieved.

4.5   TRAINING PARAMETERS

PLANNING

Plan training type and load rationally according to the amounts required by a specific discipline and by the goals to be reached in a well-defined time period. This takes place by structuring physical exercise in amounts and intensities that will provide progressively increasing workloads in order to stimulate the physiological processes of adaptation and supercompensation.

VOLUME

Volume represents the amount of work carried out during a workout unit. It is measured in different ways, according to the discipline referred to.

In bodybuilding, the total work volume is usually identified by the number of sets executed or the training session duration and by each muscle group's specific work volume (repetitions) or the time spent stimulating that same muscle.

INTENSITY

This is perhaps the most debated parameter and an object of disagreement between different schools of thought.

Definitions and formulas which are valid for performance sports aren't well suited to an anomalous discipline such as bodybuilding. In weight training, training intensity is directly related to the amount of kg [lb] lifted:

$$I = Kg\ [lb] \times R / T$$

I = Intensity
Kg [lb] = Kg [lb] lifted
R = Repetitions performed
T = Time needed to complete the set

TRAINING THEORY

This formula expresses a measure of power, since:

$$Kg\ [lb] \times R$$

merely represents Work.

The work carried out in the Time unit expresses Power, but intensity isn't simply identifiable as the measure of the power output.

Intensity is the type of effort with which a certain gesture is carried out, implying a strong subjective component which is hard to measure.

- According to Prof. Emilio They, training intensity depends on the amount of motor units involved in the unit of time between a 0-degree and a 180-degree angle (extension) or between a 180-degree and a 0-degree angle (flexion).
- Intensity is a value related to the neurophysiologic mechanism of recruitment of the various motor units, and it is not necessarily related to weight, repetitions, and duration. It is therefore a personal and contingent factor which is not measurable through external data.

Intensity in a bodybuilding exercise is given by:

$$I = IC/N \times 100$$

I = Intensity
IC = Intensity coefficient
N = Total number of repetitions performed

While executing a set, you count the number of repetitions performed from the time when real fatigue sets in. This number is the Intensity coefficient (IC). When all is taken into account, the intensity parameter is probably the most important factor in training. There is a level of intensity below which there are no biological modifications inside the muscle; it is only a waste of time.

4.6 EXERCISES

Exercises are the means of training. They are the movements through which stress is administered by applying loads to the organic levers.

Choosing the correct exercises implies evaluating their effectiveness.

Let's distinguish between complex exercises, or general conditioning exercises, and competition exercises, or specific exercises (which reproduce a specific athletic movement). In athletic training, complex exercises are used to strengthen the whole locomotor apparatus, the conditioning abilities, and motor qualities.

Competition exercises instead reproduce or imitate the technically athletic gesture typical of a sporting performance. In physical education, this concept is simplified, and we prefer to differentiate between basic exercises and complementary exercises.

4.6.1 Complex exercises

FEATURES AND FUNCTIONS

- They are multiarticular.
- They work on long kinematic chains.
- They have great muscular synergy.
- They have a straight trajectory.
- There is greater external load (lifted weight).
- There is greater internal load (the external load's effects on the body).
- There is greater recruitment of motor units.
- It has great systemic response (endocrine, lymphatic, circulatory, immune).
- It is essential for ectomorphic subjects.
- It has great hormonal response.

TRAINING THEORY

RECOMMENDED USE

- In the initial stages of fitness training (the fundamentals).
- In the general conditioning phase, where they must make up at least 70% of the training elements.
- As strength mesocycles.
- As hypertrophy mesocycles.
- During the pre-competition phase, where they must make up at least 30% of the training elements.
- In slimming programs.

4.6.2 Competition exercises

FEATURES AND FUNCTIONS

- They are monoarticular.
- They generate a pinpointed, localized, targeted stimulus.
- They have low muscular synergy.
- There is a curved trajectory.
- There is greater muscular stretching (protein synthesis increases, both *in vivo* and *in vitro*).
- There is a lower hormonal response (a slight increase in GH).
- It has qualitative movement (i.e., correct, technical movements).
- It has low synergy.

RECOMMENDED USE

- In pre-competition phase.
- As hypertrophy mesocycles.
- In overload, high-intensity techniques.
- In highly sedentary, obese, or strongly overweight subjects.
- When working on specific areas.
- In postural training.
- In physical therapy training.

Given the high organic response they create, only basic exercises truly determine the greater effectiveness of a training program. Their prevailing factor is quantitative (i.e., the load). Complementary exercises have a mainly qualitative character, especially in the course of the specific training phase. In gyms, we must distinguish between, if you will, major league and minor league complementary exercises. Let me explain: In the weights room, we don't have a technical performance objective, and it is therefore important to concentrate on those complementary exercises which yield greater muscle stretching. Stretching, both in vivo and in vitro, can in fact increase protein synthesis and induce interesting adaptations.

CHAPTER 5

FUNCTIONAL TRAINING

5.1 KINETIC AND KINEMATIC CHAINS

In human articular physiology, monoarticular movements do not exist. We could perform them, but they aren't the priority for the locomotor apparatus. For economy and practicality, our body uses complex movements almost exclusively. In physics, *kinetic chain* is a system of rigid segments connected by mobile joints called junctions.

Our body is made up of many kinetic chains that are set off by our muscles. With the term *katakinetics* (Payr[1], 1936) or *kinematic chain* (Reuleux[2], 1934), we refer to the set of organs and systems that determine the human body's voluntary movements.

- By open *kinetic chain* we mean a system in which the furthermost end (the distal end) is free and unconstrained. Example: the lower limbs when walking.
- A closed *kinetic chain* is when the distal end is fixed. In other words, it cannot move during the execution of the gesture without involving another chain. Examples: squats or horizontal bench exercises.

---

[1] Hanfried K. (2004). On the Development of the Constraint Motion Theory of Franz Reuleaux – An Overview, in *International Symposium on History of Machines and Mechanisms*, pp. 201-215.

[2] Hanfried K. (2004). On the Development of the Constraint Motion Theory of Franz Reuleaux – An Overview, in *International Symposium on History of Machines and Mechanisms*, pp. 201-215.

5.2 THE MEANING OF FUNCTIONAL

The term *functional* is very trendy nowadays, with meanings ranging from A to Z. It's like an empty tube anyone can fill up as he or she pleases with everything and nothing. Our objective is to start with a scientific definition, without which it would be impossible to build a methodology.

Let's clear any misunderstandings by working with the dictionary definition.

From the Oxford English Dictionary, Functional: of or serving a function; designed or intended to; having a function.

You can't get any clearer...

Functional training is a form of training that is related to the function for which a muscle, or rather a kinematic chain, exists and has evolved in a certain way.

The evolutionary choices of our locomotor apparatus explain the function of each muscle, kinematic chain, and articular system in our body.

How do we apply this concept?

a) by adapting it to each subject's articular structure.
b) by adapting it to the functions of the muscles or the kinematic chains which are activated.

The definition of functional training as training related to the function of the muscles in the course of a normal daily life isn't correct.

A reference parameter is actually missing: whose daily life? A weightlifting athlete's? A white-collar worker's? A sedentary person's? Daily life is different from person to person, but each one of us has the same kinematic chains.

5.3 THE ACTION-FUNCTION PRINCIPLE

The evolution in modern training is to train each muscle according to its action (a principle which is frequently applied in gyms) and to its function (a feature which is often neglected).

We must start by understanding the evolutionary choices of our locomotor apparatus.

Gyms have emphasized the concept of isolation to the extreme, focusing attention purely on muscular action but losing sight of the whole—the reason why that specific muscle, kinetic, or articular chain has evolved in a certain way.

From this stems the action-function principle:

The training of each motor feature or skill must be programmed on the basis of the action and function of the kinematic chain to which it is applied.

Without this type of programming, any training will inevitably be incomplete.

To simplify:

$$\text{Functional training } = \text{Action} + \text{Function}$$

For the same reason, functional exercises can hardly be defined as pectoralis, latissimus dorsi, or quadriceps exercises.

By working on kinematic chains as extensively as possible, large muscular areas will be engaged, even though one specific section will benefit the most.

The objective of functional training is systemic stress, involving as many organic systems as possible. This isn't enough. Understanding the evolutional changes which made us as we are today will help us understand how and why a specific muscle has developed a certain function and, consequently, how best to train it.

5.4 PEBBLES INTO A POND

Only by engaging the concept of functional training can we appreciate the shocking errors made in the development of exercises and methodologies which concentrate (often mistakenly) only on one aspect of training: action.

A few examples:

1. The femoral biceps and hamstring group

There are four muscular bands:

- Short end of the femoral biceps.
- Long end of the femoral biceps.
- Semimembranosus.
- Semitendinosus.

Of the four, only one is monoarticular: the short end of the femoral biceps. The action is flexing the lower leg to the thigh. The three others are biarticular, as they ride across the knee and hip joints. The actions are flexing the leg to the thigh and extending the thigh from the pelvis.

As stated in chapter 1, biarticular muscles must be stimulated with biarticular movements to be fully trained. In a gym there are no biarticular machines for the femoral biceps. Following the principles of biomechanics, training on the iconic leg curl machines, the only machines specific for this group, will always be incomplete.

Let's look into the function of the femoral group to discover which exercises will train it. For more information, refer to chapter 6 on the hip extensor chain.

2. The adductor group

The adductor group has three monoarticular bands and one biarticular one: the gracilis. The adductor's action is to adduct the lower limbs. The gracilis muscle adducts the thigh and flexes and medially turns the leg. The sartorius originates in the anterior part of the thigh; it is thus a part of the adductor group, but it acts synergistically with the gracilis (and with the femoral group, since it flexes the thigh to the pelvis), as flexor of the leg on the thigh.

FUNCTIONAL TRAINING

In a gym these muscles are trained, especially in women, on the classic adductor machines. Let's think about it: Do we have our evolutionary choices in mind? Monkeys, from which we derive, all have the adductor group, yet we have never seen a monkey open and close its legs in any instance in daily life. It's evident that we have lost sight of this muscle group's function, and its training is therefore incomplete. What is the adductor group's function? The adductor is a muscle with the function of acting as a stabilizer; it's also a flexor and an extensor, according to the position of its contralateral limb. It must therefore be trained with multijoint movements, using body weight.

3. Abdominal fascia: The core

This is probably the worst-trained area in the history of weight training. In gyms, core training has become a saga: a thousand and one ways of doing crunches! As with the previous point: monkeys have the abdominal fascia, as we do, but do not perform crunch movements. It's clear, then, that the abdominal fascia has other functions besides the one we train with simple abdominal floor exercises. We must not forget we are bipeds and that our customary position is, or at least ought to be, standing. If we think about it, it is intuitive that the main function of the abdominal fascia cannot be that which is performed by exercising supine on the ground. We are now ready to answer these and other questions about functional training.

5.5 OBJECTIVES

The purpose of functional training is to totally develop conditional and motor skills and motor. In simple terms, we try to train an athlete who has a propensity for strength and endurance. In other words, this athlete displays hypertrophy that isn't purely aesthetic and disappears at the first cold, but it is functional. It is useful', so our locomotor apparatus will not easily do without it.

In addition, be defined as a strength and endurance athlete, an individual must have certain body composition parameters (unless the specific performance activity directs him or her toward different weight choices). Our athlete must therefore pay attention to nutrition and supplementation. He or she must also develop various coordination abilities, beginning with proprioception (perhaps the most important one), in order to prevent injuries and optimize performance.

5.5.1 What are the benefits of functional training?

Functional training is:

More adapted to organic physiology

a) it emphasizes the relationship between the locomotor apparatus and the environment.
b) in younger subjects and particularly in older ones, it optimizes the synthesis of vitamin D (the lack of which leads to an increased risk of fractures).
c) it allows all 11 endogenous systems to activate spontaneously.
d) it takes place mostly in the standing position. How often do we forget we are bipeds? And yet, statistically, we stand for only two hours a day. Presumably the bodyweight load at the lumbar level is the main cause of back aches.

More functional

a) because you do it standing up (an athlete always ought to train standing!).
b) because it activates long kinematic chains.
c) because it trains muscular chains according to the action-function combination.
d) because it trains all of the coordination skills.
e) because it follows our evolutionary history.

More effective for training compared to the classic indoor disciplines

a)   in biomechanical terms.
b)   in muscular terms.
c)   in terms of the endogenous systems involved.

Let's just think about the difference between running on a treadmill and running on a road or dirt track.

In terms of muscular engagement, when running on a treadmill we do have the eccentric phase of the movement but the concentric phase—the extension of the thigh on the pelvis—is performed by the treadmill's own rotation, partially blocking the full motion of the gluteus. Furthermore, the foot strike is cushioned by the machine. The simple impact of the foot on the ground (not necessarily bumpy or unpaved) during a run or a walk outdoors has magnified consequences from a biomechanical point of view, and it also trains proprioception.

Also consider the work done using a road bike or a mountain bike compared to that done in a gym on vertical or horizontal stationary bikes.

5.6 MOTIVATIONS

The objective of functional training is to create athletes, forming our bodies into personalized outfits.

Another outcome of functional training makes it unique. Our motivation to become more fit on the outside goes hand in hand with improvements at the physical level. The more a person appreciates the progress and the strengthening of the organic systems (cardiorespiratory, endocrine, lymphatic, musculotendinous), the more that person will become mentally stronger, more determined, motivated and efficient. He or she will train in increasingly demanding conditions (rain, cold weather), with increasingly more intense activities (uphill and downhill running exercises, forest exercises).

Whoever said that functional, body-weight exercises are easy? Challenge yourselves on dirt tracks, beaches, meadows, or any other outdoor or indoor surface. Execute walking lunges for only 100 m (109.4 yd) because it doesn't matter how long you take; you can stop, rest, catch your breath...and then carry on!

Three days or a week later, return to the "scene of crime" and do the same exercise, but try one of three things differently:

1. Cover the same distance in a shorter time.
2. Take the same time but increase the distance covered.
3. Take less time and increase the distance.

Trying is believing!

5.7 FUNCTIONAL TRAINING AND PRE-ATHLETICISM

The term *pre-athleticism* can have two meanings:

1. Development of the athletic components in a child during the growth phase.
2. Training for specific performance sports.

And even a third new meaning, the one we refer to, about generic pre-athleticism or general physical preparation (GPP):

3. Multilateral work structured for the development of motor and coordinative abilities functional to a general psycho–physical enhancement.

In terms of this, Hirtz's[3] (1985) model identifies seven coordinative abilities:

1. Kinesthetic differentiation ability.
2. Movement combination and segmental coordination ability.
3. Reaction ability.
4. Orientation ability.
5. Balancing ability.
6. Adaptation and transformation ability.
7. Rhythmic ability.

To these general abilities we can add three others:

8. Motor learning ability.
9. Movement control ability.
10. Movement variation ability.

GPP work is, for the majority of athletes, the secret for working functionally and for wearing one's body like a dress.

Functional training will allow you to climb the steps of physical efficiency, while at the same time developing all those qualities which constitute the basis for it.

---

[3] Hirtz P. (1985). *Coordination Abilities in School Sports*. Volk und Wissen.

TRAINING WITH KETTLEBELLS FOR STRENGTH AND MOBILITY

5.8 FUNCTIONAL TRAINING: OTHER FACTORS TO DEVELOP

5.8.1 Training recruitment

Training recruitment means working on the central nervous system. The best age to obtain established improvements in this sense is before 14; specific training beyond this age will, however, improve several factors in recruitment, both spatial and temporal, though with a semi-automatic acquisition.

EXAMPLE 1

A child learns to ski and then, for whatever reason, doesn't practice this activity for a few years. When the child puts the skis back on, he or she will ski as well as before stopping (it will only be necessary to reacquire confidence).

EXAMPLE 2

An adult learns to ski with perseverance and frequency then, for whatever reason, doesn't practice for years. When the adult puts the skis back on, he or she will have to start almost from the beginning again (the stoppage time factor is significant).

Let's distinguish between spatial and temporal recruitment:

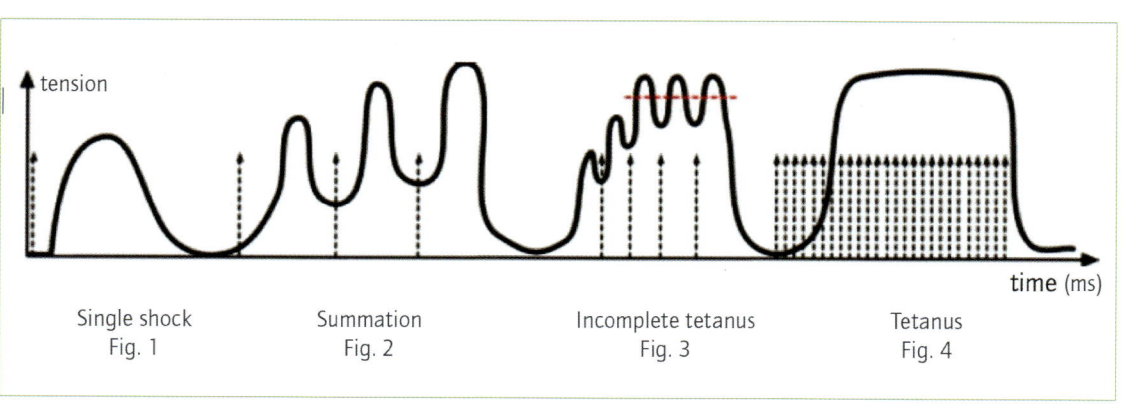

Summation

FUNCTIONAL TRAINING

- **Spatial recruitment:** it is the increase in the number of motor units recruited during contraction and can be one of two types:

1. *progressive:* strength is developed gradually along the time scale (imagine pressing the foot down gradually on a car accelerator).
2. *ballistic:* the command signal reaches the muscle in a tiny window of approximately 100 ms (Paillard, 1982). Imagine flooring the accelerator immediately and hard.

- **Temporal recruitment:** it's the increase in the discharge frequency by the nervous system (via summation).

  - When a motor signal is sent by the central nervous system to a single fiber, the fiber first contracts then releases (fig. 1).
  - When the motor message is transmitted more effectively by increasing the impulse frequency, the tension generated by the muscle increases through the summation effect of two closely-spaced impulses (fig. 2).
  - With several closely-spaced impulses, the tension produced will increase further as a result of their summation, the clonus condition (fig. 3).
  - Beyond this limit, if the impulse frequency increases still, the maximum possible tension, called the tetanus, is developed (fig. 4).

5.8.1.1 Training recruitment in adults

It is possible to train the central nervous system, hence training recruitment, in adults. The objective is to increase neuromuscular activation by performing exercises outside the usual criteria:

- **More complex exercises:** involving long chains and working with several body districts together in order to force the central nervous system to engage in a higher effort.
- *Uncomfortable, destabilizing exercises:* using unconventional or differentiated equipment, making the execution more difficult; working from a standing position with differentiated loads, involving the body's stabilizing systems and muscles.

- **Plyometric and isometric contractions:** alternate to the normal concentric and eccentric phases. Varying the type of contraction within the same exercise has an uncommon training impact.
- **Working on the muscle's elastic components:** with exercises which involve a pre-stretching of the muscle trained (i.e., pulling away its origin and insertion). We forget that working with these factors is inside us—it is part of primitive activities such as running, walking, jumping, and sprinting.
- **Functional exercises:** training the muscles according to the action-function principle.

5.8.2 Strengthening pivot muscles

Whatever its objectives, training must reinforce pivot muscles for preventative and also performance improvement purposes. By pivot we mean those muscle groups belonging mainly to the deep musculature with the main function of joint stabilization—muscles which are loaded with tension during exercise performance.

The main ones are:

- Rotator cuff
- Flexors and extensors of the forearm and fingers
- Periscapular muscles
- Wide abdominal muscles
- Paravertebral muscles
- Tibial and adductor muscles
- Triceps surae muscle

When building an athlete, training these groups must take precedence over training others.

FUNCTIONAL TRAINING

5.8.3 Reinforcing the weak links in the kinematic chains

It is of utmost importance when training to remember in a kinematic chain, the weakest muscle influences the functionality of the entire chain. If we have a chain made of several iron links and one paper link, the paper link will be the first to give way, and because of its frailty, will weaken the whole chain. Working on kinematic chains allows us to examine the weakest muscular links and to work on strengthening them using

- chains,
- elastics bands,
- kettlebells,
- sandbags,
- medicine balls, and
- shortened movements with supports.

Contrary to common wisdom, work on the weak link should not be aimed at hypertrophy. We must always take into account the synergy of the muscles involved in the same chain.

5.8.4 Breaking the pattern

This is one of the most interesting aspects of functional training: the ability to progress in a thousand different directions, to apply a variety of stimuli which gym activity cannot provide. Any structure, any object, whether natural or not—a tree, a branch, a rock, a rising slope, a flight of steps, a sand or cement sack, a wood, a beach, a track, a meadow, a dirt track, a low wall—can become the center of new workouts, new exercises, or new applications of the same.

The first step in breaking the pattern and building a motor map as wide as possible is to stimulate the central nervous system with basic exercise programs and unconventional exercises—the key principle being movement variation. And change an exercise not session by session but set by set, within the same session.

TRAINING WITH KETTLEBELLS FOR STRENGTH AND MOBILITY

Every time we subject our central nervous system (and consequently the locomotor apparatus) to a new type of movement, we apply stress to it. At this stage, the central nervous system will be forced to adapt and enhance all the systems involved, owing to the continuity and repetition of the movement. A body which is prodded by multiple stimuli will be always proactive, ready to change; it will be able to react and adapt much more quickly. Variability of movement is the central nervous system's oil (Guido Veestagen[4], 2014).

As an example of what we mean, let's describe an exercise and its progression set by set:

1. Walking lunge.
2. Asymmetric walking lunge (weight on one arm only).
3. Walking lunge with two dumbbells.
4. Overhead walking lunge (one arm lifts the weight above the head).

Working on long kinematic chains, for example, is almost unknown in gyms, excepting squats and deadlifts. These are typical weightlifting technical gestures in which, after the loading phase, the weight is heaved upward and the body is simultaneously lowered in the opposite direction, fitting underneath the load. They are extremely difficult for the average gym patron, who is used to heavy loads but extremely simple exercises.

---

[4] Veestagen G., (2010-2012-2014). Personal communication, *Perform Better Convention*, LA.

CHAPTER 6

TRAINING WITH KETTLEBELLS FOR STRENGTH AND MOBILITY

6.1   PRESENTATION

Ask any athletics coach from Eastern European countries or the US: "Where does the secret of strength lie? Where does it come from?" They will reply: "From the hips, from the hip extensor chain". Hip muscles express strength and power more so than other muscles. It is not a coincidence part of the hip extensor chain is the gluteus, the human body's strongest muscle (after the masseter, the chewing muscle). Think of any performance sport and you will see that in some way this chain is deeply involved in it.

HIP EXTENSOR CHAIN

Training the lower limbs has a great importance in terms of prevention and pre-athleticism, even more than aesthetics. Studies provide ample confirmation of this when training is supported by basic exercises. Let's start with what we know: Ample articular excursions in the lower limbs (i.e., full squats) determine significant hormonal distress (Bosco[1] and coll., 1996).

It is clear then: the lower limb training bastions (squats, leg presses, sagittal lunges, deadlifts) do work. Their combined use satisfies any and all needs for strength, tone, and muscular tropism. But the question we must ask ourselves is: do they train thighs and glutes completely? The answer is no! These exercises actually train the gluteus, the quadriceps, and in general the lower limb muscles according to their action and the flexion and extension of the thigh on the pelvis, but not their function.

Do we remember the concept of functional training? It is Action + Function. What is the function of the gluteus? It is propulsion.

Now take a look around gyms, and you will notice that there are no exercises featuring propulsion or that work with propulsion in any way.

In the training this chain, exercises in which this thrusting action is present are missing, such as

- jumps,
- skips,.
- plyometric jumps,
- uphill walking,
- sprinting (better if uphill),
- starter exercises,
- swing exercises, and
- ballistic exercises.

Functional training = Action + Function

Let's never forget it.

---

1 Bosco C. and Viru A. (1996) *Biologia dell'allenamento*, SSS, Roma

6.2 ACTION AND FUNCTION OF THE LOWER BODY

The function of the coxofemoral joint and of the muscles which originate or are inserted nearby confirm the necessity for functional training of the lower body.

The muscles in the joints of the lower body contrast the effect of gravity and of any other force that tends to destabilize the body's balance.

The functions of the lower-body muscles are:

- Double support in the upright stance.
- Oscillation and support during locomotion.
- Transfer of the body from a lying down to an upright position.
- Sensitive information from the support points.

During ambulation, when one leg is lifted, the hip muscles are active in shifting the body weight onto the support limb and preventing the pelvis from falling down the side which isn't supported.

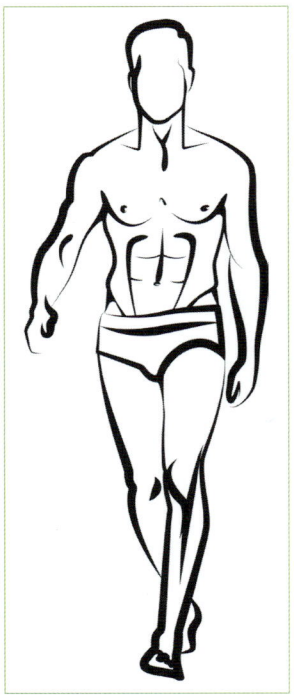

ADDUCTORS

They contract to shift the pelvis toward the support side; furthermore, they can act as hip extensors or flexors when walking or running, according to whether they are forward or behind the rotation axis. Finally, they stabilize the pelvis.

ABDUCTORS

When walking and running, they stabilize the pelvis on the support side, preventing it from falling.

ILIOPSOAS

It rotates the pelvis forward and is active in walking, climbing stairs, running or walking uphill, and getting up from a supine position.

HIP EXTENSOR CHAIN

QUADRICEPS

When running, it helps the gluteus to realize its maximal potential in the final extension phase.

GLUTEUS MAXIMUS

It is the body's most powerful muscle, the largest (66 cm2 [25.9 in2] in section) and the strongest. Its main action is the extension of the thigh on the pelvis. Its function is propulsion. This muscle is indispensable when running, jumping, and marching uphill.

FEMORAL BICEPS, SEMITENDINOSUS, AND SEMIMEMBRANOSUS

The femoral muscle group had already been reevaluated by the athletic training schools in Eastern European countries, and these evaluations are shared by American athletics coaches. It is a group of biarticular muscles (except for the short end of the femoral biceps), that ride the knee joint distally and the coxofemoral joint proximately. As such, their main action is the extension of the thigh on the pelvis, in synergy with the gluteus maximus, to which they also offer a great functional support in propulsion.

PIRIFORMIS MUSCLE

It is a hip abductor. Its action is maximized at a 60-degree flexion of the hip. It has an external rotation action before reaching 60degrees of flexion and an internal rotation one beyond 60 degrees. Pivoting on the femur, the piriformis inclines the pelvis contralaterally and tilts it backward. The piriformis is important because of its close contact with the sciatic nerve. Symptoms such as sciatic pains similar to those found in cases of herniated discs are frequent and attributed to an excessive shortening of this small muscle; curiously, they are also called "wallet-in-the-back-pocket syndrome", since the habit of wearing such objects seems to lead to articular compression and the shortening of the piriformis.

From this we can deduce that the main action of the coxofemoral joint and therefore of the whole hip extensor chain is propulsion. In order for the training of this kinematic chain to be complete, then, following the action-function principle, we have to add to basic and multijoint exercises of proven effectiveness (e.g., squats and lunges) and other exercises in which this function is expressed.

TRAINING WITH KETTLEBELLS FOR STRENGTH AND MOBILITY

6.3 ARTICULAR REALITY: LONG-LIMBED AND SHORT-LIMBED SUBJECTS

We said at the beginning that articular reality, which varies from individual to individual, is an expression of functionality and therefore of evolutionary choices.

Among articular systems, the coxofemoral is the one that most exemplifies this evolution. Anthropologists have in fact noted how the shape of the femur—diaphysis, neck, and head—responds exactly to these evolutionary criteria. Its shape is variable and depends on functional adjustments. We can therefore distinguish two different types: the long-limbed subject and the short-limbed subject (Bellugue, P., 1963).

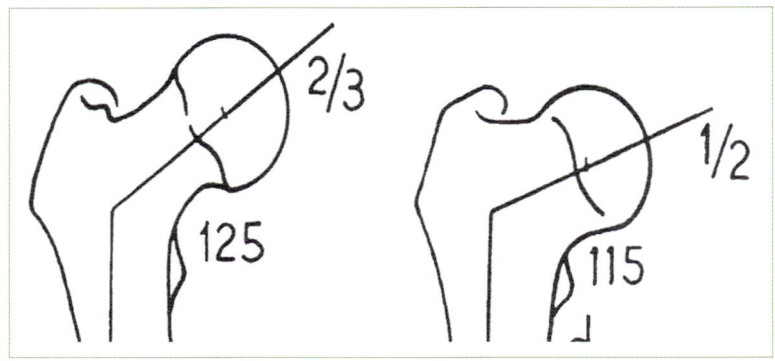

Femur head in long-limbed and short-limbed subjects (picture from Kapandji).

LONG-LIMBED TYPE

The femur head is a sphere 4-5 cm [1.5-1.8 in] in diameter for more than two thirds of the femur, supported by the femur neck which binds it to the diaphysis.

The femur neck axis forms with its diaphysial axis a tilt angle of 125 degrees and a declination angle of 25 degrees with the frontal plane.

The femoral diaphysis is thin, and the pelvis is small and high. This combination means a wide articular excursion of the femur head within the articular cavity, and this ensures great articular width, which can mean a talent for running. This subject is therefore suited to this type of activity (think of the Kenyan marathon runners).

HIP EXTENSOR CHAIN

SHORT-LIMBED TYPE

The femur head is barely larger than a half of a sphere; the tilt angle of the femur neck corresponds to 115 degrees, while the declination angle is about 10 degrees. The femoral diaphysis is short and thick. This combination means a limited amount of femur head excursion within its articular cavity. It is a morphology of strength. What the subject loses in terms of speed, he or she regains in strength and power.

6.3.1 Consequences

A specific anthropometric trait corresponds to a characteristic biotype.

Without dwelling too much on this, when we talk about biotype (from the Greek *bios* and *tupos*, meaning life print), we mean a group of individuals with similar physical, hormonal, personality, and other features. **The long-limbed type,** also called ectomorphs, is only slightly hypertrophic in both upper and lower body. It is an adrenaline-sensitive subject, with high levels of catecholamines and thyroid hormones and low levels of testosterone and androgens. It is poorly suited for weight training and tires easily and quickly.

Ectomorphic, mesomorphic, endomorphic.

Training for this subject will need to be exclusively focused on long kinematic chains, involving large muscular areas; the training ought to incorporate the classic basic exercises and functional movements that are expressions of strength and power (skips, vertical and plyometric jumps, one-legged jumps). This is because we need to induce a strong hormonal response, especially at the androgen level, through training.

The short-limbed type, endomorph, has a greater propensity to upper- and lower-body hypertrophy. Generally, it has a low metabolism, great muscular mass and strength but also a propensity to gain weight. The female subject will have to pace herself in the basic exercises and include functional movements with aspects of endurance (uphill walking or walking) that do not involve white fibers. The male subject will easily increase muscular mass and will have to concentrate on slimming. A typical training program could feature one day of total body weights, one or two of circuit training, and possibly one day exclusively dedicated to aerobic work.

6.4 BACK ACHE, THE ILIOPSOAS, AND EVOLUTION

Evolutionary choices form the basis of functional training and explain the adaptations and changes our body has gone through in the course of millennia. What we are today is the result of those choices. What is amusing is that we never think of ourselves as an outcome. So to speak, 6.5 million years ago we were a bunch of Australopithecines. The achievement of the upright posture is supposed to date back to about 2.5 million years ago. It represented a huge leap along the evolutionary scale. To explain this better: The life of an anthropomorphic monkey takes place over 10 square miles, while our hominid ancestor could cover this distance in just one day when hunting for food. Then followed the reversal of mandibular prognathism.

Coming to the present age, it is clear that evolutionary choices have always had biological and physiological justifications (we are, after all, the dominant species on the planet). We must proceed from here and think about the current issues. The most common pathologies in bone and joint muscular terms are back pains, especially at the sacral-lumbar level. The vertebrae that are statistically most affected are L5-S1 and L4-L5. At the heart of these aches there is almost always an excessive retraction of the hip flexors. The shortening of the iliopsoas—and even more common in sporting subjects, of the rectus femoris—is responsible for a more or less pronounced hyperlordosis; this attitude is favored by hypotonia of the rectus abdominis. The number one cause of these retractions is a sedentary life. Look at small children, and you will notice that they execute perfect squats with complete ease, and they easily hold a full crouch. Similar adaptations are still to be found today in several people on various continents. We have forgotten that man has evolved as a biped and as such must functionally discharge tensions and loads to the ground through a system of joints and shock absorbers: the joint capsules. The problem is that today, so statistics say, we stand up for only two hours a day and for the rest of the time we sit down on chairs, stools, seats, and sofas. A sedentary lifestyle doesn't fit with the evolutionary processes, albeit only progressively in older subjects. In all of these non-physiological positions, the support point for the locomotor apparatus is the pelvis in the sacral area. This is where we discharge forces and tensions for eight, ten, and even more hours every day, causing neuromuscular retractions as well. We could then ask why our body has chosen to preserve the iliopsoas despite all the problems it causes. We know that it is an important muscle for walking and running, according to Delmas' spinal index, but this feature has become more pronounced after coming down from the trees.

What about before? Why was it already there before? What is the function of the iliopsoas? We can use the following example to find the answer. A young man in a gym is performing chin-ups. For the first few repetitions, it all goes well; the body is perpendicular to the ground, and the execution is correct. Then fatigue sets in. What does our subject do? He bends the thighs into the pelvis. Why? Because in doing so he shortens the lever's arm and manages to complete a few more repetitions. Monkeys, from which we descended, execute the same movement when they move from one branch to another: They stretch and extend in the aerial phase, and shorten themselves by flexing their thighs and trunk during the traction phase. Also, when chimpanzees walk, they lean forward with their trunks and diminish the lordosis of their lower backs. Remember that the psoas muscle creates lordosis in the back by arching it. Monkeys keep using the iliopsoas, but they start from a lengthening position. Probably humankind has not yet adapted to the upright posture, and this would explain the dichotomy between the psoas function on the one hand and the use we make of it on the other. In general, seeing the difference between their action-function and current use, I believe it is always best to train these muscles by stretching them.

CHAPTER 7

7.1   PRESENTATION

When we talk about the abdominal fascia, we are discussing the most important area for the health of the bone-joint apparatus. The relevance of this whole area has come increasingly more important so that you frequently hear about core training. The abdominal segment connects the trunk and the lower limbs. The lumbar-pelvic region consists of:

- 35 bilateral muscles inserted in the pelvis.
- 14 muscles that link the pelvis to the spine.
- 21 muscles that connect the pelvis to the lower extremities.

ABDOMINAL FASCIA

The abdominal corset (picture from Kapandji[1]).

In the course of evolution, the rachis has changed from being a link between upper, anterior limbs and lower, posterior limbs to an antigravity support structure with static and dynamic features. In the presence of hypotonia of the rachis musculature, we assume incorrect and deficient postures which may lead to spine problems, such as postural defects, or pathologies, such as hyperlordosis, hyperkyfosis, or worse, scoliosis. A strong athlete will have a strong abdomen and toned, efficient abdominal fascia.

---

1 Kapandji I.A (1983). *The Physiology of the Joints*, Elsevier Churchill Livingstone Publisher.

7.2 CORE

The functions of the abdominal fascia are stabilization, motion, and control. But we are specifically talking about these muscles:

- Rectus abdominis
- Transversus abdominis.
- Internal oblique muscles.
- External oblique muscles.
- Quadratus lumborum.
- Erector spinae.
- Pelvic floor muscles.

We may think of the core as a bucket. The cylindrical supporting structure consists of three strata of muscles: the transversus abdominis and the oblique muscles. The anterior securing hinge is the rectus abdominis, and the posterior hinge is made of the erector spinae muscles and the quadratus lumborum. The bottom of the bucket is made by the pelvic floor muscles.

7.3 PELVIC FLOOR

The pelvic floor is a group of muscles which creates a weave among the pelvis bones. In the course of evolution, with the shift from a horizontal, quadrupedal or semi-quadrupedal posture to the upright posture, the pelvic floor muscles have decidedly changed their function. If before their almost exclusive function was waste expulsion and synergy in parturition, now with the bipedal posture they have acquired the role of support platform for the organs and the abdominal cavity. In the female subject, the poor activation of pelvic floor muscles is the cause of frequent pathologies, especially post-childbirth complications, from incontinence to the prolapse (a collapse) of the uterus.

7.4 ACTION OF THE ABDOMINAL FASCIA

The core's complexity relates primarily to its muscles.

RECTUS ABDOMINIS

This muscle flexes the trunk forward and laterally; it raises the pelvis and participates in abdominal pressure. It plays an important role in maintaining the correct posture of the pelvis, as an antagonist to the quadratus lumborum. It is a muscle with an important aesthetic value, but, functionally speaking, it is secondary to the large abdominal muscles.

EXTERNAL OBLIQUE MUSCLE

This muscle is synergistic to the rectus abdominis in the flexing of the trunk. It tilts the trunk laterally and turns it contralaterally (the right external oblique muscle turns the trunk to the left, and vice versa). It participates in the final rotation extension in all the throwing movements practiced in athletics such as rugby, tennis, baseball, golf, and even boxing. Every time we apply a weight to one side of the body (e.g., carrying a suitcase or a dumbbell), the oblique muscles on the opposite side contract in order to stabilize the trunk and prevent it from falling laterally. It is part of the abdominal corset.

INTERNAL OBLIQUE MUSCLE

This muscle shares in the forward flexion of the trunk; it tilts the trunk laterally or turns it toward the contracting side. In rotation, it is synergistic with the rectus abdominis and the external oblique muscle on the opposite side. It contributes to abdominal pressure.

TRANSVERSUS ABDOMINIS

This muscle's main activity is abdominal pressure: It holds back the viscera and stabilizes the pelvis. It is thanks to the synergy between the transversus abdominis and the oblique muscles that the pelvis and the lumbar tract acquire strength and stability.

QUADRATUS LUMBORUM

As the name itself suggests (*quadratus* means "square" in Latin), this is a square-shaped muscle that goes from the iliac crest to the spine and the ribs. It tilts the trunk backward and laterally. It is the real antagonist of the rectus abdominis.

ERECTOR SPINAE AND LATISSIMUS DORSI

Their action is the extension and lateral tilt of the back.

7.5 FUNCTION OF THE ABDOMINAL FASCIA

Let's start talking about the function of the abdominal fascia muscles beginning from the synergy between the diaphragmatic and the mediastinal cavities that border each other. They are physically divided but functionally associated. With inspiration, when the thorax expands, the mediastinal cavity is depressed; with expiration it is the diaphragmatic cavity which is depressed, while the mediastinal cavity expands. Endo-abdominal or peritoneal pressure increases during an effort, especially when it is combined with forced expiration (Zatsiorskij and Sazonov[2], 1988). As a result of the internal support, pressure on intervertebral discs may be reduced by 40%; it is produced by the activity of the abdominal wall, intercostal, and diaphragm muscles.

*The pelvis
(picture taken from Kapandji[3]).*

The picture of the pelvis (from Kapandji) reproduces a cutaway of the mediastinal cavity from which the action of the large muscles of the abdomen is evident: the external oblique, the internal oblique, and the transversus abdominis. These three muscles warp the abdominal cavity in three superimposed circles, joining at the front in a fibrous aponeurosis, into the weave in which the rectus abdominis is inserted. This already shows us that it is almost useless to work on the rectus abdominis to reduce the waistline because it doesn't have much influence. For this purpose we ought instead to focus on the three previously mentioned muscles. The abdominal fascia function as:

---

2 Zatsiorskij V.M. and Sazonov V.P. (1988). "Basi biomeccaniche nella prevenzione dei danni alla colonna lombare durante esercizio fisico - Revisione della bibliografia esistente", in *Atleticastudi*, 5.

3 Kapandji I.A (1983). *The Physiology of the Joints*, Elsevier Churchill Livingstone Publisher.

- **Stabilizers.**

Their role in containing the viscera and as stabilizers is ensured by isometric contractions which set the pelvis in an anatomic position. Let's think about it: If the erect posture is, or ought to be, the one most frequently adopted, our abdomen's number one function cannot be that of flexing the trunk on the ground, as with crunches and similar exercises, but rather it is the stabilization and rotation of the pelvis, working against gravity (does anyone do these exercises in gyms?).

- **Motors.**

The dynamic function is guaranteed by anisometric contractions of those muscles which allow flexion, lateral flexion, and rotation of the trunk and lifting of the pelvis. Once again we are not talking about one single muscle but about a functional, synergistic set. The majority of these movements still takes place in the upright position. If we think about trunk rotation, we realize that the first and most frequent gesture of this type happens when walking.

- **Respiratory mechanisms.**

The abdominal fascia contribute to expiration and, in particular, to forced expiration. The latter is produced by the activity of the abdominal wall muscles, the intercostal muscles, and the diaphragm. In many sports where there are expressions of strength and power, it is a virtually physiological activation.

The visual and aesthetic effects of good abdominal corset firmness, and specifically firmness of the transversus abdominis, are several.

The firmer the transversus abdominis, the thinner the waistline is, since there is an accent on the curve which delimits it laterally and which coincides with the area between the ribs and the pelvis: the hip line (hyperboloid line). A firm abdominal corset implies a series of benefits, the most important being:

- Less stress on the lumbar rachis.
- Greater core strength owing to the action of the pivot muscles.
- Reduction of back pains, owing to the increased stabilizing function.
- Reduced visceral ptosis.
- Improved synergy between lower and upper limbs in the work of kinematic chains.

7.6 THE CENTRIFUGE PRINCIPLE

In training theory, the core's importance is confirmed by its first-place ranking in the sequence of muscular areas to be trained in beginners: the centrifuge principle. This because the abdominal fascia and the joints which rely on it are the fulcrum upon which the forces coming from the upper body and the stress coming from the lower limbs (impact with the ground) are discharged. It is not by chance that the rachis is the area most subject to wear and to inflammatory pathologies: back pains, sciatica, and lumbago. And it is no less by chance that the back pains of 50-year-olds are becoming a heritage of the younger generations.

CHAPTER 8

SCAPULOHUMERAL GIRDLE

8.1 PRESENTATION

Only functional training allows us to determine instances of contradictions in our locomotor apparatus.

The scapulohumeral joint is a case in point. It is an enarthrosis, like the coxofemoral joint. In other words, it has a greater range of movement compared to other joints.

Unlike the coxofemoral joint, however, where trunk weight contributes to the stabilization of the femur head within its articular cavity, in the scapulohumeral joint, the humerus is simply hanging from the trunk. In fact, when the deltoid muscle is at the point of maximum contraction with the arm abducted at 90 degrees, the humerus head deviates from the line of articular constraint.

The conformation of the shoulder joint tells us that our bodies' evolutionary choice has been one of mobility at the expense of stability.

The humerus head, in fact, only partially adheres to the glenoid cavity, remaining mostly outside the articular constraint.

Rather than entering the glenoid cavity, the humerus hangs from the trunk and moves in different directions. It is able to do this because of its active stability, created by the development of the nearby musculature, and its passive stability, ensured by the same muscles' tendons and by the ligaments.

Besides the scapula stabilizers, the only muscles with a prevailingly stabilizing function are those in the rotator cuff, a real articular reinforcement structure.

Question: Don't you find it strange that all the muscles richest in white fibers are inserted on the most unstable joint in the human body?

- Triceps long head: 67% of white fibers.
- Trapezius: 64% of white fibers.
- Latissimus dorsi and pectoralis muscle: 50-58% of white fibers.
- Deltoid (anterior, medial, posterior): 40% of white fibers, located chiefly in the anterior part.

Yet white fibers tell of high workloads, expressions of strength and power, and great tension. On a joint that is unstable? Almost as a confirmation of this, anyone who has trained the scapulohumeral girdle muscles intensely, though correctly and without overdoing it, has been virtually obliged to suffer through painful and inflammatory pain in this joint. Why such problems? Where do they stem from? Read the next paragraph, and you will find the answer.

8.2 ACTION OF THE SCAPULOHUMERAL GIRDLE

All the muscles involved in the movements of the shoulder region are distally inserted on the humerus, scapula, and clavicle. These three bone segments share everything.

TRAPEZIUS

The upper band plays an important role in all traction and lifting movements; it lifts the shoulder and rotates the scapula. The medial band retracts the shoulders, bringing them closer to the spine.

The lower band rotates the scapula and depresses the shoulder in synergy with the pectoralis minor muscle. Besides, when contracted unilaterally, the trapezius rotates the head laterally. We notice it when we have irritating neck problems, in which the contracture of the trapezius or the sternocleidomastoid heightens the pains associated with them.

DELTOID

This is a powerful abductor of the upper arm. It can raise the arm above the head. The clavicular bands lift the arm forward; the acromion bands lift it up laterally; and the scapular bands abduct the arm backward.

Besides, it has an active stabilizing role for the joint, which it covers like a cap.

It is activated in arm circumduction movements typical of swimming and boxing.

It works in synergy with the pectoralis major muscle in all pushing movements along different planes.

PECTORALIS MUSCLE

It works in synergy with the deltoid's clavicular bands in order to flex the shoulder at 90 degrees.

It adducts and intrarotates the shoulder, flexing the arm on the transverse plane.

SCAPULOHUMERAL GIRDLE

With arms raised and fixed, it pulls the trunk upward (the climber's movement). In all suspension and support movements, it prevents the lowering of the trunk together with the latissimus dorsi. It is also active in the forward lifting of the arm from the outside back position (discus throw) and from the below back position (bowling). It cooperates in deep breathing. The synergy of the pectoralis with the triceps is extremely important in explosive, fast pushing movements (i.e., sweeping aside branches and twigs). The long head of the triceps is in fact statistically the muscle with the highest percentage of white fibers.

LATISSIMUS DORSI

It is dedicated to the extension, adduction, and internal rotation of the shoulder joint. In all suspension and support movements it contributes to the stabilization of the trunk. It forcefully lowers an elevated limb (e.g., in throwing or hitting movements). It also pulls the trunk toward the arms. As we can see, it performs many movements in synergy with the pectoralis, to which it is often and wrongly considered antagonist. (How can two muscles with the same distal insertion, both acting as intrarotators of the humerus, be antagonists?) When the hand is above the head, the latissimus dorsi pulls the arm down and backward against the resistance, as if we were lowering a portcullis. In a climbing action, the hand is placed above the head, and the latissimus dorsi works hard to pull the trunk toward the arms, lifting the whole body upward. In subjects with a functional lower-body functional deficit, if it is impossible to lift the body from a seated position by extending the lower legs, the hands can lean on the chair's armrests and push and lift the body up, exploiting the adduction action of the latissimus dorsi as it lifts the pelvis. When walking on crutches, the latissimus dorsi helps the hands bear the body's weight (see how monkeys walk).

SERRATUS ANTERIOR MUSCLE

Its action consists of pulling the scapula forward around the thorax (protraction). This movement increases the ability to stretch the upper limb forward, adding strength to the gesture of hitting with a fist or overcoming a resistance ahead (i.e., sweeping asides leaves and branches).

TRICEPS

This muscle has both biarticular and monoarticular features. Its long end, which is biarticular, acts as extensor of the forearm on the arm and as extensor of the arm on the trunk. It helps the pectoralis major and the deltoid in extensions and thrusts, and it helps the latissimus dorsi as it retracts and adducts the arm.

It is the antagonist of the biceps and the muscle responsible for the largest part of the arm's volume.

BRACHIAL BICEPS

This is another biarticular muscle. Can you then explain to me why I often see it trained with the elbows blocked alongside the trunk, with a monoarticular movement? The biceps' proximal segment is covered by the deltoid and the pectoralis major. The biceps is a flexor of the forearm and of the humerus; it is also a supinator of the forearm. When the elbow is extended, the biceps tenses to contrast the force of gravity. It also acts as a help to the latissimus dorsi in tractions.

8.3 FUNCTION OF THE SCAPULOHUMERAL GIRDLE

What is the function of the shoulder joints?

As we have seen, the scapulohumeral girdle is an extremely complex crossroad of muscles, tendons, articular systems, and a kinematic chain that is the victim of an apparent incongruity. Yet it is simple: The scapulohumeral girdle is a transducer of forces, a functional hub. Exactly like a rail hub, purpose of the shoulder joints is to transmit the forces coming from the lower body or the trunk to the upper body.

The scapulohumeral girdle's function suggests exercises and execution modes different from those used now and in the past. It tells us, for example, that there is a contraindication to training the deltoid with a load applied to the uper limb only (e.g., slow forward movement and slow barbells) without the help of the lower chains. It also tells us that we cannot ask for stability with excessive movement control and slow-motion executions from a joint that doesn't have this feature. It is better to train it with exercises in which the thrusting action starts from the lower body and, with their help, is then transmitted to the upper body via the scapulohumeral joint. Exercise examples include: push-press exercises with dumbbells or barbells and jerk, clean, and press exercises. Paradoxically, training requires much higher loads for a shorter timeframe. This is what this articular systems demands. Actually, if you think about it, any sporting activity featuring a transmission of forces from the lower to the upper part of the body, such as boxing, baseball, tennis, golf, weightlifting, or martial arts, follows this line. You will enjoy greater results in terms of strength and hypertrophy, and pains, inflammations, sub-acromion syndromes, and contrasting syndromes will decrease or even disappear.

8.4 GRIP TYPES

Grip is an issue which is seldom discussed in gyms. It is generally thought to be a factor of secondary importance. However, there comes a time in training when the subject starts adopting a personalized grip, often based on unorthodox suggestions (the most common is: "use this grip, you'll feel the pectoralis better"). Actually, strength stems from the grip. Power grips bring the maximum amount of the sensitive area of the fingers and the palm of the hand in contact with the object being gripped. The four fingers flex around the object while the thumb wraps around the opposite side; this way the sensitive receptors of the areas involved ensure there is the right pressure for controlling the barbell. In this action, all the muscles in the fingers and thumb that close the hand are active: the muscles of the thenar eminence and the hypothenar stabilize the palm's medial side against the object, the finger muscles grab, and the wrist extensors impart a stable base to the gripping action. Pay attention to when you close your fist; notice the hand, wrist, and forearm become one single functional block, a single segment. The harder the hand grips an object, the greater the wrist extensors' activity is and the more extensive the central nervous system's motor signal is. One of the primary reflexes in a newborn baby is flexing the fingers when pressure is exerted on the center of their palm. This kind of grip and the physiological reactions which subsequently intervene increases nerve response and muscular fibers recruitment.

SCAPULOHUMERAL GIRDLE

CHAPTER 9

TIBIAL-TARSAL JOINT AND FOOT

9.1 PRESENTATION

The peculiarity of the foot is that it is the only part of the human body in continuous contact with the ground. While the vast majority of animals stand and ambulate on their fingers (digitigrade), man is a plantigrade (i.e., he or she rests the whole sole of the foot on the ground). When we stand, the ground exercises a force which is equal to and opposite to our body weight called ground reaction force. This and other forces are applied to the inferior limb joints—pelvis, knee, and ankles—which for this reason have a very high functional synergy. The role of the foot and ankle joints is:

- To orient the foot in order to set the sole correctly on the ground.
- To modify the shape and curvature of the plantar arch in order to adapt the foot to the ground's asperities and to create a system of shock absorbers between the ground and the leg.

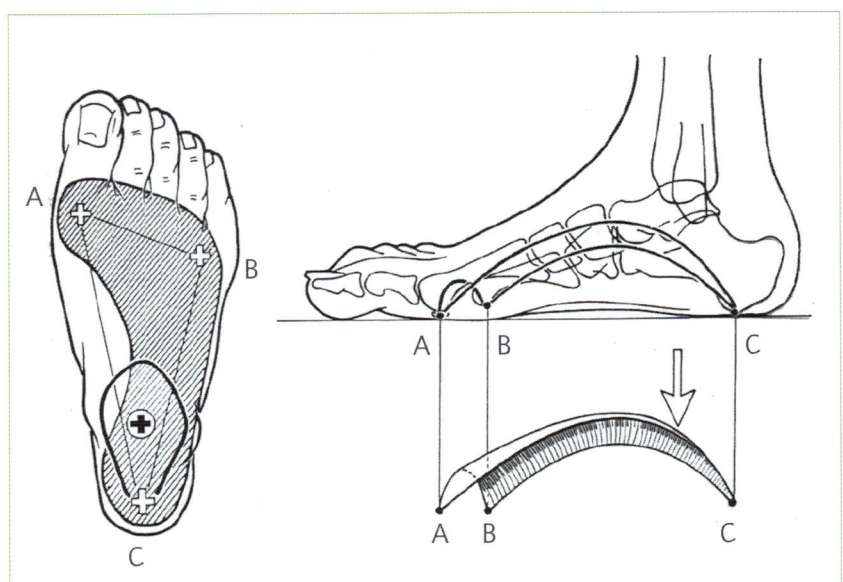

The foot (picture taken from Kapandji[1]).

---

[1] Kapandji I.A (1983). *The Physiology of the Joints*, Elsevier Churchill Livingstone Publisher.

9.2　WALKING

In terms of the tibial-tarsal joint, the posterior tibial, gastrocnemius, and soleus are the muscles chiefly responsible for propulsion when walking, running, and jumping. The action of the calf muscles is augmented by arching the foot and flexing the toes. When the heel leaves the ground, the toes extend, increasing the plantar arch. Walking is technically like a fall cushioned by the contralateral limb. In ambulation, we have a foot-plant phase for approximately 60% of the stride and an oscillation phase, with the foot off the ground, for about 40%. This means there is an alternation of monopedal support and bipedal support phases. At the start of the foot-plant phase, the foot is forward of the trunk and pushes ahead and toward the ground, decelerating the body's fall and providing support. In the final phase, though, the foot is at the rear of the body and pushes down and backward, providing acceleration. Let me underline the intervention of the upper body in ensuring a correct, coordinated posture as a confirmation of our physiological conformation based on kinematic chains.

TIBIAL-TARSAL JOINT AND FOOT

9.3 RUNNING

When running, the percentage ratios change drastically: the foot-plant phase ranges between 40 and 27%, depending on speed .The faster the athlete is, the shorter the ground foot-plant phase will be (sprinters reach about 22%).

Running efficiency is the result of the accumulation and release of potential energy within the elastic component of the tendons and of the energy-transfer action by the muscles that stretch across the lower joints. The kinematic chain activated by the running action sets off and involves initially both the gastrocnemius and the soleus. Both muscles help the action of the plantar arches and the forefoot. Then, in sequence, it involves the quadriceps, the hip extensor chain (femoral biceps and gluteus), and the abductors, compensating for the pelvis' fall at the foot plant. In terms of the foot, the action of the astragalus is essential. This is the bone that partitions the forces applied by the ankle and the tibia during the various phases. Because of the action of the plantar arches and the ligaments which run across the foot, the foot functions as a spring, ensuring the return of 80% of the elastic energy.

9.4 FOOT MOVEMENTS

As we have emphasized before, functional training points in one direction: training based on kinematic chains, following the evolutionary lines of the human race. It also suggests a different approach for gyms and sports centers: The action and function of a muscle, or a kinematic chain, should never be separated. We cannot disregard dynamic movements when training the musculature that runs across the tibial–tarsal joint, especially the triceps surae.

Let's think about it. These bone–joint structures have evolved for walking and running, and as such they have always been subjected to propulsive forces, both acceleration and deceleration. The exercises usually performed in gyms, even on machines, do not consider these features. It is a serious mistake to constrain our articular systems, which vary from individual to individual, by training only by the rectilinear path imposed by a machine. We have also seen how there is a synergy between the triceps surae and other muscles of the leg and thigh. It is obvious they have to be trained together in order to avoid a regression in terms of intra- and intermuscular coordination.

PART II – PRACTICE

CHAPTER 10

10.1 PRESENTATION

10.1.1 Origins

The origins of kettlebells are lost in the mists of time. We find them mentioned officially for the first time in a Russian dictionary of 1704. Their first use takes us to the markets on the Persian border, in Asia Minor; the kettlebell was the weight used in commercial scales. In those parts, where different peoples and cultures met to exchange, buy, and barter housewares and fine fabrics, the unit of measure was the *pood*, equivalent to about 35 lb (16 kg). Merchants boasted they could manage to put 2 or 3 *pood* of weight in kettlebells on the scale's plate to counterbalance the equivalent weight of the goods exchanged. It is told that Tsar Alexander III saved his life and that of his family in a railway accident thanks to the strength he had acquired, so he claimed, training with his beloved *giryas* (Russian word for kettlebells). From that moment on he made the use of kettlebells during PE lessons compulsory in schools. In more recent times, a former *Spetsnatz* officer, Pavel Tsatsouline, brought kettlebells to the US and from there use of this weight began to spread like wildfire.

10.1.2 Introduction

You either love or hate kettlebells. Sometimes both. I was lucky to get started on my way to becoming a kettlebell master with two great tutors: Steve Cotter and Ken Blackburn, the chairman and v-chairman of the International Kettlebell and Fitness Federation (IKFF); both were tutors at the RKC, Pavel's school in Paris, before leaving it. I continued my professional development with *girya* sport multi-world champion, Oleh Ilika. Each one of them—especially Steve, who honors me with his friendship—has given me much both in technical and human terms, and I am deeply grateful to them for this. When you share the same passions, it doesn't take long to become friends. You simply acknowledge each other.

The most shocking error about kettlebells is the conviction, on the part of some people, of having the universal technique, the only technique possible. Nothing could be farther from the truth. I leave this presumption to others, and I prefer to reason with my own head. The more arrows I have in my bow, the better I will be armed and ready for any event… or won't I?

I know at least 20 different types of swing and, over time, for different types of fitness training, they have all been useful to me. I don't like to sell hot air, so the exercises contained in this book will not be the same, with one exception maybe, as those included in my previous book on this theme (*Kettlebell*, Elika Publishers). Just to make an example, we shall work with kettlebells in unconventional ways, too.

TRAINING WITH KETTLEBELLS FOR STRENGTH AND MOBILITY

10.2 LOWER-BODY EXERCISES

KETTLEBELL DEADLIFT

Starting position

- **A |** Sit back into a half-squat, with the legs bent as if you were about to jump up. The back is arched, following the spine's physiological curves, with the chest forward and the scapulae closed.
Extend your arms and grip the kettlebell, which is lying on the ground, level with your heels.

Execution

- **B |** Keeping the scapulae together, extend the pelvis up and forward until you rise to a standing position.

KETTLEBELL EXERCISES

- **C |** Slowly return down, bringing the pelvis backward, and sit back into a squat again.

C

Discussion

The kettlebell deadlift is a great exercise, with both limitations and merits. Compared to its "older brother" with the barbell, its limit is the load, which is inferior, and the narrow grip, which, since it prevents a correct retraction of the scapulae in the lifting phase, tends to unbalance the body forward, bringing the shoulders forward. The merit is in the range of the movement, which is much deeper and fuller. The barbell is in fact placed against the tibiae, while the kettlebell goes well beyond them, toward the heels. This way you achieve a greater stretching of the hip extensor chain and a greater activation of the elastic components of the muscles related to it. It is a very interesting movement, the more so since the load issue is partially resolved by the evolution of the exercise, the two-kettlebell deadlift (not described here). It is a must for developing iron glutes, femoral muscles, erector spinae, and parascapular muscles. It's recommended for all.

TRAINING WITH KETTLEBELLS FOR STRENGTH AND MOBILITY

TWO-ARM SWING

Starting position

I recommend two ways of starting out: one for those people (k-bellers) who are already familiar with kettlebells, and one for those who still haven't had the chance to become familiar with this exerciser (beginners).

- **A |** K-bellers: sit back into a half-squat with the kettlebell lying on the ground between your feet, the back in the neutral position (with physiological curves activated), and the head aligned with the spine, looking toward a point forward on the ground.

- **B |** Beginners: stand with the kettlebell just below the pelvis, the arms relaxed.

Discussion

Number one! This is my judgment on this swing. It is a ballistic exercise, and as such—we have already said so but it never hurts to repeat it—it subverts Henneman's[1] recruitment law, activating pure white fibers (or fast-twitch or type IIx fibers) immediately. This feature makes it essential for athletic training but also for fitness

---

[1] Henneman E., Somjen G., and Carpenter DO. (1965). "Functional significance of cell size in spinal motoneurons", in Journal of Neurophysiology, 28: 560-580. – Henneman E. and Olson CB. (1965). "Relations between structure and function in the design of skeletal muscles", in Journal of Neurophysiology, 28: 581-598. – Henneman E, Somjen G, and Carpenter DO. (1965). "Excitability and inhibitability of motoneurons of different sizes", in Journal of Neurophysiology, 28: 599-620.

KETTLEBELL EXERCISES

Execution

The swing is like a jump without leaving the ground.

- **C |** Flex the pelvis back and wind up the hips, bringing the kettlebell just below the pelvis. The legs are slightly bent, the knees almost stationary, and the back still in the neutral position.

- **D |** Extend the hips explosively and, exploiting their momentum, swing the kettlebell up in front of you. The arms can be slightly bent or straight; the kettlebell's flat part is parallel or slightly below an imaginary wall placed in front of you.

or bodybuilding programs. The swing teaches the activation of the coxofemoral joint and of the muscles related to it: the glutes, femoral, and hamstring muscles. Also, the swing activates the pelvis and trunk stabilizers, the longissimus dorsi, oblique, rectus abdominis, quadratus lumborum, and pelvic floor muscles, as well as the trapezius and parascapular muscles. It also stimulates the cardiovascular and cardiorespiratory systems. It is an essential exercise for training for women, too. Circle in red, and respect!

TRAINING WITH KETTLEBELLS FOR STRENGTH AND MOBILITY

BOX SQUAT

Starting position

- **A |** Adopt the rack position: Stand upright, about 4 in. (10 cm) in front of two steps, with the arms and forearms close to the trunk and the kettlebells closing the arm–forearm triangle.

Discussion

This exercise is a must according to many American fitness coaches. The reason is simple. Like the swing, the box squat trains the hip and back extensor chain activation, albeit in a different fashion. It is a preparatory exercise and a waypoint necessary for strength conditioning with heavier loads. The image you should picture in your mind during the execution is that of sitting down on a chair which is progressively being snatched away from behind you. After placing yourself 4 in. (10 cm) from the steps (a stool or a bench will also do), the first step is to bring back the pelvis and immediately afterward bend the legs; the back is arched (emphasize the spine's curve slightly, without exaggerating) so as to activate the paravertebral and parascapular muscles. Right from the start you can feel the activation of the gluteus and of the femoral group, as well as the quadratus lumborum and the spine

KETTLEBELL EXERCISES

Execution

- **B |** Holding the kettlebells close to the torso, flex the pelvis backward and bend the legs until you are sitting on the steps. Straighten your pelvis and legs and stand up again.

extensor muscles. In this exercise, the progression can take different directions. You should evaluate and choose them according to the subject:

- Increase the load (you may also use a barbell).
- Increase the movement's depth by sitting down on boxes or stools or steps that are progressively lower.
- Increase the movement's width by moving farther away from the steps.

The exercise is particularly suitable for women, because in the rising phase it strongly activates the gluteus and allows the use of weights (which are essential for an optimal work on this muscle) in absolute safety. I personally regard it as a required exercise.

TRAINING WITH KETTLEBELLS FOR STRENGTH AND MOBILITY

OVERHEAD SQUAT

Starting position

- **A |** Stand and raise the kettlebells above your head. You are in the lockout position: The arms are close to your head, held straight and slightly intrarotated, and the thumbs are diagonal to the head.

Discussion

This is an overhead exercise, and that says it all. Sink into a maximum squat without lifting the heels and maintaining the spine's physiological curves—this is important. Always keep the arms raised overhead. The degree of activation of the back extensor musculature and of the parascapular muscles is high, and this makes the overhead squat another must for athletic training in any sport that features propulsion (running, sprinting, jumping, kicking) and also a waypoint for strength and power mesocycles. Beginners will start with the simplest execution and then follow the exercise's progression:

KETTLEBELL EXERCISES

Execution

- **B |** Without changing the arms' position, flex the pelvis backward and bend the legs until you sit back into a full squat.
Slowly return to the starting position and complete the required repetitions.

- Body-weight squats with only one arm overhead.
- Squats with both arms overhead (deep squats).
- Squats with only one overhead arm and an added weight.
- Overhead squats.

In a sedentary subject, such a progression is not possible from one day to the next, but this is the route to follow.

119

TRAINING WITH KETTLEBELLS FOR STRENGTH AND MOBILITY

OVERHEAD WALKING LUNGE

Starting position

- **A |** Stand and hold one kettlebell in each hand. Leave the left arm loose at your side and bring the right arm overhead into the lockout position.

Execution

- **B |** Take a step forward with the left leg.
- **C |** Lower the right knee, as though you were kneeling down.

KETTLEBELL EXERCISES

- **D |** Push up and forward, advancing with the right leg.
- **E |** Lower the left knee, as though you were kneeling down. Repeat the sequence and complete the required repetitions, switching the overhead arm set after set.

Discussion

The overhead walking lunge is the functional exercise par excellence for the lower body. Do you remember action + function? It has everything: flexion–extension (i.e., action of the gluteus-femoral-quadriceps chain) and propulsion (i.e., function of the hip extensor chain). To these stimuli let's add, in terms of exercise, the overhead work, which is exceptional from a postural point of view, because it trains the whole paravertebral musculature: the parascapular and trapezius muscles and the rotator cuff. The overhead walking lunge is also an excellent core workout, because it trains the entire abdominal fascia. The asymmetric load distribution ensures that the internal and external oblique muscles are strongly engaged to stabilize the pelvis and torso. For all sports which feature a synergistic activation of lower and upper body, this exercise must—I repeat, must—be a part of the training program.

TRAINING WITH KETTLEBELLS FOR STRENGTH AND MOBILITY

STEP SNATCH

Starting position

- **A |** Sit down on two steps (you can also use a bench or a stool). Regulate the height of these supports so that the pelvis is slightly below the knees.
  The right hand grips the kettlebell and intrarotates (the palm of the hand faces the body). The kettlebell is lying on the ground next to the supports.

Discussion

No ballistic exercise is as effective as the snatch in terms of the forces it generates: acceleration, explosiveness, strength, balance, and stability. Also, the cardiovascular, musculotendinous, endocrine, and immune systems are all involved. This cocktail makes it a unique exercise for general conditioning. The step snatch is used to increase the strength and power of the hip extensor chain. The muscles which rest on the coxofemoral joint—gluteus, femoral muscles, hamstring, and quadriceps—and with

KETTLEBELL EXERCISES

Execution

- **B |** Extend the hips with a fast, explosive movement of the gluteus (the force imparted will depend on the load lifted). Propelled by the hip thrust, continue moving the kettlebell up. The arm holding the kettlebell is slightly flexed so as not to overload the elbow joint and to fully complete the technique.

When you are standing, immediately extend the arm, imagining you are punching up. You are now in the lockout position.

Bring the kettlebell back down with the arm in the rack position.

Sit down on the steps and set the kettlebell on the ground.

Complete the required repetitions required, and then repeat with the other arm.

B

them all the muscles that support back and upper-body extension must express strength and power (which translates into acceleration) from rest, without the ballistic wind-up they are used to. This is a fantastic exercise, ideal for all those sports which involve jumps or major expressions of power, such as rugby, American football, wrestling, volleyball, beach volleyball, MMA, combat arts, basketball, and skiing. Circle in red, and respect!

TRAINING WITH KETTLEBELLS FOR STRENGTH AND MOBILITY

SQUAT AND PRESS

Starting position

- **A |** Stand holding two kettlebells in the rack position: The arms are resting on the sides, the forearms next to each other, and the two kettlebells closing the two triangles between arm and forearm.

Execution

- **B |** Keeping the arms in contact with the trunk, bend the legs and sit back into a full squat.

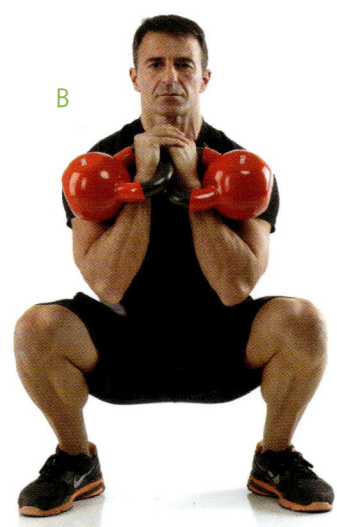

Discussion

How I love this exercise! It is absolutely functional. The majority of performance sports requires synergy between lower and upper body. If you pay attention, you will see that this type of movement is most difficult for those who train in gyms. They are used to extremely simplified exercises, pushed by the obsession with working on the muscle and not on the gesture. Let me remind you that our central nervous system does not reason in terms of individual muscles, but in terms of gestures (i.e.,

- **C |** Rise up explosively, extending the legs. Use the lower-body propulsion to lift the kettlebells above your head; the thumbs are diagonal to the head (the right thumb points to the left ear and the left thumb to the right ear). Bring the kettlebells back into the rack position and complete the required repetitions.

in terms of the synergy between muscular chains). This is what weightlifters do and is the reason why Olympic lifts are extraordinary athletic training exercises—not just for expressions of strength. The squat and press trains the synergy between lower body, core, and upper body. The thrust (propulsion) starts from the hip extensor chain during the ascending phase of the squat. From here it is transmitted to the abdominal fascia and from this to the upper body. The scapulohumeral joint system works in a fully functional way, as a conductor of forces: great loads in a small time frame. It is an excellent exercise for combat arts, martial arts, boxing, rugby, American football, basketball ,and volleyball. Circle in red twice.

WINDMILL

Starting position

- **A |** Stand and hold a kettlebell with your right hand. Bring the right arm into the lockout position; the other kettlebell is on the ground next to the left foot.

Execution

- **B |** Maintaining the lockout position, turn the feet diagonally to the left.

Discussion

Few exercises are as fine to watch and are felt so strongly as the windmill. And few exercises are as effective. Hip extensors, abdominal fascia, quadratus lumborum, erector spinae, longissimus dorsi, rhomboid, trapezius, parascapular muscles, deltoid, triceps, and rotator cuff are all involved.

KETTLEBELL EXERCISES

- **C |** Looking at the kettlebell above your head, push the right hip laterally and back while at the same time leaning laterally and down to the left, trying to keep the legs as straight as possible. Grasp the kettlebell lying on the ground with the left arm.

- **D |** Pivoting on the right hip, lift the torso slowly until you return to the upright position, and complete the required repetitions. Finally, switch the starting arm to execute the movement on the other side.

The muscular chain which gets activated is truly significant. The frontal plane of movement, as well as the transverse one through the torso's rotation, are little used in traditional exercises. Even as a body-weight exercise, this is perfect for soccer players, sedentary people, and all those with a blocked tibial-tarsal and coxofemoral joint, with the ensuing retraction of the muscular chains which are inserted there. I like it. Circle it in red!

GET-UP PRESS

Starting position

- **A |** Sit down on the ground, with the left leg extended in front of the body and the right leg bent; the torso is upright.
Grip the kettlebell with the right hand and hold it in the rack position, placing the left hand on the ground for support.

Execution

- **B |** Extend hips and pelvis explosively upward, exploiting the hip propulsion to lift the kettlebell.

KETTLEBELL EXERCISES

- **C |** Return to the ground with pelvis and glutes, bringing the kettlebell back into the rack position. Complete the required repetitions. Switch the position of the legs and repeat the exercise on the other side.

C

Discussion

This is another unconventional and extremely effective exercise. The abdominal fascia doesn't have a stabilizing function alone, as was believed until not long ago, but also a motor function which in turns conducts forces to the upper body. This is one of the exercises which trains the core in this skill. Another interesting factor is the press movement exercised in both directions by the arm which lifts the kettlebell and by the arm resting on the ground, with an intense involvement of the humerus and scapula stabilizer muscles and the latissimus dorsi. Gray Cook includes it in his rehab protocols specifically to engender this type of action. The hip extensor chain action should not be underestimated.

TRAINING WITH KETTLEBELLS FOR STRENGTH AND MOBILITY

ONE-LEG KETTLEBELL DEADLIFT

Starting position

- **A |** Stand and lift the right leg slightly; the arms are at the sides and the kettlebell on the ground in front of you.
  Pause to gain balance and stability before starting the exercise.

- **B |** Lower the torso slowly downward and grip the kettlebell with the right hand.

- **C |** With a controlled movement, lift both torso and kettlebell, returning to the upright position. Keep your balance without setting the right leg on the ground, and complete the required repetitions.

KETTLEBELL EXERCISES

- **D and E |** Switch both the support leg and the arm that grasps the kettlebell, and execute the exercise again for the same number of repetitions.

Discussion

This is a fantastic exercise—one of the few which trains whole-body extension—and the absolute best for gluteus and femoral muscles. Let's not forget the work to which the spine's extensor muscles, the quadratus lumborum, longissimus dorsi, erector spinae, humerus retractor muscle, and extrarotator cuffs, are subjected. In addition, it features balance, proprioception, and destabilization, all essential conditions in performance sports. Important: Always keep the spine in the neutral position. The one-leg deadlift must be taught gradually. My advice is to start by asking your pupil to simply touch the kettlebell that lies on the ground and to return upright without lifting it. The next step is to touch two kettlebells placed in front of the legs with both hands. The third step is the exercise described here. The fourth progression involves lifting two kettlebells with both hands. An extra progression of this exercise is the one-leg deadlift executed from on top of a step, with the kettlebell lying on the ground.

KETTLEBELL ALTERNATE-STEP DEADLIFT

Starting position

- **A |** Stand on top of two steps, placed about 12 in. (30 cm) apart. The kettlebell is on the ground between the two steps.

Execution

- **B |** Bend your legs and sit back into a full squat.
  Grip the kettlebell with your right hand and lift it, returning to the standing position.
  Squat down again.
  Pass the kettlebell to the left hand.
  Stand up again.
  Repeat, alternating the hands during lifts, and complete the required repetitions.

Discussion

This exercise has been devised for a deep movement and a full range of motion. The hip extensor chain is more stimulated than in the normal execution without steps so that gluteus, femoral muscles, and quadriceps work flat out. And there is more. The alternately monolateral weight, in other words, the destabilization on both sides, engages the pelvis and hips stabilizers as well as the whole adductors group: the gracilis muscle, the gluteus minimus and medius, and the abdominal fascia. Let's not forget the work of the whole paravertebral musculature—the quadratus lumborum, erector spinae, trapezius, parascapular muscles, rhomboid, and extrarotator cuff muscles. Asymmetric work has been rediscovered in training programs. The training inputs and the effects on training transfers are unique. This is an exercise that influences athletic performance.

TRAINING WITH KETTLEBELLS FOR STRENGTH AND MOBILITY

10.3 CORE TRAINING

KETTLEBELL SIT-UP

Starting position

- **A |** Lie supine on the ground and hold the kettlebell with the right hand with the right arm extended. Keep the left arm diagonally on the ground.

Discussion

I usually talk about the features of an exercise. Here I do the opposite. I start from what the exercise is not, as a necessary introduction to prevent, or at least dampen, the criticism by those training puritans who will probably snub their noses at this execution: "Did you check the posture?" "Does the back remain in the neutral position?" (These are typical questions they may pose). The kettlebell sit-up isn't an exercise for beginners, it isn't advisable for everyone, and it isn't even an exercise to be performed with regularity and frequency in training. On the contrary, it must be included for short periods and planned for gradually and carefully within athletic training. Why should you include it then? And when? Virtually no performance sport follows the rules of correct posture or biomechanics.

KETTLEBELL EXERCISES

Execution

- **B |** Plant the heels on the ground and, keeping the kettlebell overhead, raise the torso rapidly. Stop when the torso is perpendicular to the ground and the right arm is in the lockout position.
Return to the ground slowly and controlled. Make sure that the back is in the C curve. Complete the required repetitions and then repeat, switching the hand that holds the kettlebell.

None is good for the joints. Whether we like it or not, this is the reality. How many times, when teaching lunges, we say that the perpendicular line drawn from the upper knee must not go beyond the foot's tip in order not to overload the knee joint? Have you seen the lunges of fencing athletes? They go well beyond that! How many times do we warn against stressing the scapulohumeral joint excessively? Have you seen the cross at the hoops? Frightening tensions! This is the reality we have to deal with. The kettlebell sit-up is recommended for all those sports where there are strong and often unforeseen stimuli to the whole abdominal fascia—hits, tackles, and tearing movements, for example. It is ideal for martial arts, combat arts, MMA, tennis, rugby, American football, basketball, baseball, and powerlifting. If included gradually, it is a great exercise.

TRAINING WITH KETTLEBELLS FOR STRENGTH AND MOBILITY

DOUBLE KETTLEBELL SIT-UP

Starting position

- A | Lie supine on the ground. Hold a kettlebell in each hand and extend the arms straight up.

Execution

- B | Plant your heels on the ground and, keeping the kettlebell overhead, raise the torso rapidly.

  Stop when the torso is perpendicular to the ground.

  Try to keep the arms extended and bring the head forward, looking up toward the kettlebells.

  Return to the ground slowly and controlled, resting the back on the ground in the C curve. Complete the required repetitions.

Discussion

The same that was said for the previous exercise is the same for this exercise. If I had to choose between the two, I would be really undecided. Sit-ups with two kettlebells requires you to manage a heavier load, though performing them with only one kettlebell has, as extra input, greater destabilization. The double kettlebell sit-up engages the rectus abdominis specifically, whereas if you use only one kettlebell, you activate the oblique muscles more. They are both excellent exercises, however, which you can include and plan for in the athletic training for the sports mentioned previously.

KETTLEBELL EXERCISES

ROLL-UP, ROLL-DOWN

Starting position

- **A |** Stand in front of a mat. Hold a kettlebell in your hands, keeping the arms close to the torso.

Execution

- **B |** Bend the legs and sit back into a deep squat.

  Squat down farther until the glutes and the pelvis are resting on the mat behind you.

  Roll back, as if you wanted to perform a roll, and at the same time straighten the arms (and the kettlebell) back beyond your head. Once you reach the movement's limit, when the speed decreases, invert your direction, almost executing a forward roll.

  Straighten the arms in front of your torso and, exploiting the wind-up's speed, step up on your feet.

  Lower down again and repeat.

Discussion

Very fine, very comprehensive: The adjectives are suitable but they aren't sufficient to define this absolutely unique exercise. Coordination, integration, multiplanar work; hip and torso extensor chain, abdominal fascia. What more do you want? How you manage the weight, a kettlebell, or another exercise tool is also interesting. In the first and second parts of the movement—the squat and the backward half-roll—the weight acts as extra resistance for the agonist muscles. In the third and fourth parts—the forward half-roll and stepping up to the standing position with arms straight—the weight is a facilitating factor. At that moment, the body is like a scale, and the weight it carries in the direction opposite to the body is a load which is subtracted from the body's weight. This is an excellent exercise for free wrestling, MMA, martial and combat arts, rugby, American football, and basketball.

HOT POTATO

Starting position

- **A |** Sit down on the ground, with the legs flexed.
  Hold a kettlebell in your hands using the goblet grip: The hands are wrapped around the kettlebell, not the handle.
  Gather your arms into the chest.

Execution

- **B |** Lift your feet, supporting yourself on the buttocks.
  Keeping the kettlebell in the center of your torso, start rotating the chest to the right and left.
  Complete the sequence for the number of repetitions or the time required.

Discussion

Pretty much the same that was said for the kettlebell sit-ups is the case for the hot potato. This is actually a comprehensive exercise which stimulates the whole core: the rectus abdominis, the oblique muscles, the quadratus lumborum, and erector spinae. The problem could lie in the equally high activation of the rectus abdominis, the psoas, and the hip flexors. It is a fair criticism, and I accept it. However, competitive sports require performance, not correct posture or biomechanics, and athletic training must necessarily conform to this, because of its preparatory role. I have used this exercise very often in fitness plans for fight and contact sports—full contact karate, Thai boxing, wrestling, MMA, rugby, American football, baseball, and basketball—and also for other sports where the same articular systems are likewise stimulated: tennis, motocross, motorcycle racing, and mountain biking. It is a worthwhile exercise.

KETTLEBELL EXERCISES

KETTLEBELL REVERSE CRUNCH

Starting position

- A | Lie supine on the ground, the knees bend and the feet on the ground. Raise your hands behind the head and grip two kettlebells placed on the ground behind you.

Execution

- B | Keeping them flexed, raise the legs and bring the calves in contact with the thighs. Exhaling, lift the pelvis with a controlled movement, bringing the knees toward the chest.
Inhaling, bring the legs and pelvis back down slowly.
Complete the required repetitions or perform for the preset time.

Discussion

The reverse crunch is one of the few crunch exercises I still favor. I have already explained the reason—it is functional training. Crunch exercises aren't functional, even though we can modify and improve them by positioning a rope beneath the lumbar area. At any rate, I believe that the reverse crunch is more physiological compared to the normal crunch, because it recalls ancestral movements which have been part of our history. In this case, the two kettlebells make the exercise easier compared to the body-weight execution, because you can use them to anchor your upper body.

TRAINING WITH KETTLEBELLS FOR STRENGTH AND MOBILITY

KETTLEBELL SWING WITH ROTATION

Starting position

- **A |** As for the normal swing, I will suggest two ways to start, one for k-bellers who are already familiar with kettlebells, and one for those who aren't familiar this exerciser yet (beginners).

- **B |** *K-bellers:* in the crouch position, the kettlebell is on the ground between the feet; the back is in the neutral position (the physiological curves are activated); the head, aligned with the spine, looks toward a point ahead and below you.
Beginners: stand with the kettlebell just below the pelvis, arms relaxed.

Execution

- **C |** Flex the pelvis back and, winding up the hips, bring the kettlebell back (the kettlebell is just below the pelvis; the lower legs are slightly flexed; the knees are almost stationary; and the back is in the neutral position).

Extend the hips explosively and, using their propulsion, swing the kettlebell forward and up (the arms may be straight or slightly bent; the kettlebell's flat part is set parallel or slightly below an imaginary wall in front of you).

Immediately afterward, pivot on the left forefoot and turn the torso to the right, shifting the kettlebell's trajectory not to the center but to the right (the kettlebell follows the hip movement).

Return to the wind-up phase and complete the required repetitions.

Repeat the exercise, pivoting on the right leg and rotating the torso to the left.

Discussion

This exercise requires coordination, strength, resistance, balance, and proprioception. To the beneficial effects of the swing you add rotation work on the transverse plane, a must for all sports. Baseball, judo, wrestling, MMA, combat and martial arts, basketball, soccer, tennis, volleyball, rugby, American football: Can any sporting activity do without training rotation movements? No. This exercise still needs to be discovered in terms of potentialities and additional effects. Performed to a preset time and with a significant load (one step at a time, please), it has exceptional aesthetic and physiological effects. I don't know any other exercise among all those I have listed that can train rotation so effectively. Perform it, and you will realize this, too.

TRAINING WITH KETTLEBELLS FOR STRENGTH AND MOBILITY

10.4 UPPER-BODY EXERCISES

PUSH PRESS

Starting position

- **A |** Stand holding two kettlebells in the rack position: The arms are hugging the sides, the forearms are close to the torso, and the two kettlebells close the triangle between arm and forearm.

Execution

- **B |** Keeping the kettlebell in the rack position, bend the knees rapidly with a short movement.

Discussion

This is a functional training exercise *par excellence*. If executed well, the greatest part of the effort will be borne by the hip extensor chain and not by the arms or the deltoid muscles. Training the synergy and coordination between the hip extensor chain and the upper body is the best solution to improve performance in sports in which this combination is essential, such as boxing, basketball, volleyball,

KETTLEBELL EXERCISES

- **C |** Extend the legs explosively, assisting the torso's movement with the upper body, and raise the arms up, putting the kettlebells into the lockout position (the arms are extended up and are close to the head).

- **D |** Bring the kettlebells back into the rack position, flexing the legs slightly to cushion the impact.

combat and martial arts, rugby, and American football. When we see a boxer fighting with heavy arms and having difficulty throwing punches, this is because the hip activation has stopped, and the effort falls entirely on the arms—a job too costly for such small muscles or kinematic chains. The paradox is that, compared to ordinary gym exercises for the shoulders, arms block, with this push press you will use much heavier loads and will become even stronger, tougher, and more powerful, with far fewer risks. Circle it in red.

TRAINING WITH KETTLEBELLS FOR STRENGTH AND MOBILITY

BENT PRESS

Starting position

- **A |** Hold the kettlebell in the right hand by the right shoulder. Imagine you are wearing a backpack on your right shoulder:
Bend the legs slightly.
Rotate the tips of your feet diagonally to the left.
Lean laterally with your torso until your left hand reaches the left knee.
Shift the right hip laterally and back. The hip is the real supporting pillar of the movement.

Discussion

Those who know me are aware that I have a weakness for this exercise to the point that I get excited when I talk about it and demonstrate it in seminars. The bent press is a legendary exercise. 19th-century and early 20th-century strongmen believed it was the basis for a muscular, harmonious body. Some myths suggest that Arthur Saxon or Eugene Sandow (immortalized in the Mr. Olympia statuette) recommended it as the first exercise to practice. As I wrote in *Kettlebell* (Elika Publishers),

KETTLEBELL EXERCISES

- **B |** Push the right hip back. Lean laterally and down with the torso while at the same time pressing the kettlebell up. The arm holding the kettlebell is perpendicular to the ground, and the left hand is on the ground.

it remains a mystery to me why such an effective exercise, with few contraindications, should have been progressively abandoned and supplanted by other exercises that are less effective. Personally, I regard it as the best lifting exercise for the upper body. No extension can be as comprehensive, and no technique engages the whole musculature of the trunk so fully and intensely. Extension, rotation, involvement of the lower body: It has everything! This exercise is the basis for any strength training. Once you overcome the dejection after the initial learning phases of the technique, if you keep training, the bent press will repay the time you spent a hundredfold. It is excellent for all those sports featuring expressions of strength, power, explosiveness, and hip, torso, and scapulohumeral girdle rotations: throwing sports, judo, martial and combat arts, baseball, basketball, rugby, golf, tennis, volleyball, water polo...there are none excluded.

TRAINING WITH KETTLEBELLS FOR STRENGTH AND MOBILITY

FLOOR PRESS

Starting position

- **A |** Lie supine on the ground, with the legs flexed and the feet on the ground. Hold a kettlebell in each hand, keeping the arms in contact with the floor and the forearms perpendicular to the ground.

Execution

- **B |** Push the pelvis up and align the body like a diagonal plank, supporting yourself on the scapulae. Stabilize the position. Push the arms up, lifting the kettlebells above your chest. Keep the pelvis in an elevated position and start performing a set of presses with the arms only.

KETTLEBELL EXERCISES

- **C |** Return to the starting position and repeat.

Discussion

This exercise is highly underestimated. Criticism to it derives from the fact that in the eccentric phase (in other words, the descent) the arm touches the ground before the pectoralis muscle reaches maximum stretching. This could cancel, at least partially, the effectiveness of the exercise. I don't agree with this opinion Here's why. First of all, in gyms we frequently use the barbell when we do bench presses. This is an exercise tool which limits the arms' range of movement because of its very shape. You stop the movement when the barbell rests on your chest, though the arms could finish well below it (as happens with dumbbells). This isn't the core of the issue though. Let's take a look at the position and the kinematic chains involved:

- The lower limbs, gluteus, adductors, abdominal fascia, paravertebral muscles, trapezius, parascapular muscles, and extrarotator cuff muscles are all isometrically activated with a stabilizing function.
- The pectoralis-deltoid-triceps block works dynamically against a resistance which is very different from what is offered by a barbell or a dumbbell. The kettlebell, owing to its physical shape, is a destabilized weight, and as such it doesn't feature de-tension points through the arc of its movement.

At the point of maximum contraction of the pectoralis, with the hands intrarotated and the arms extended over the chest, the shortening is greater than that obtained with a bench press; the effect and perceived weight are greater than those produced by dumbbells of equal weight. The floor press is therefore an outstanding exercise you can add to other gym classics, and it is also the first step toward the step floor press. This is an exercise in which you place both feet and scapulae on two separate steps, working on the depth of the movement and achieving maximum stretching of all the bone and muscular systems activated. Trying is believing!

RENEGADE ROW

Starting position

- **A |** Adopt the push-up position with hands on two kettlebells and straighten the body like a plank. The feet are resting on the ground, the arms straight, the hands grip the kettlebells, and the shoulders are perpendicular to the hands.

Execution

- **B |** Keep the body stable, concentrating on the alignment of pelvis and trunk. Then lift the kettlebell with the left arm, holding the arm close to the torso. Be sure to not rotate the pelvis or the trunk.

KETTLEBELL EXERCISES

- **C and D |** Get back down slowly and repeat the movement with the right arm. Complete the required repetitions.

Discussion

This is a great exercise. It is usually listed as an exercise for the latissimus dorsi, but this is just the tip of the iceberg, because the whole abdominal fascia is totally involved. The core works constantly to stabilize the pelvis and further activate further the oblique muscles every time the arm that lifts the kettlebell changes. The latissimus dorsi works dynamically with the arm that lifts the kettlebell and works isometrically, together with the pectoralis, with the arm that acts as ground support and carries the weight of the whole trunk. This is a truly comprehensive exercise, the basis for athletic training in all those sports in which the core is subjected to great tensions, such as combat sports, martial arts, wrestling, judo, rugby, American football, tennis, and baseball.

LONG-CYCLE CLEAN AND PRESS

Starting position

- **A |** Hold a kettlebell in each hand and stand with your arms in front of the hips.

Execution

Start in the same way as in the swing. Imagine a jump with no aerial phase.

- **B |** Flex the pelvis back and wind up the hips; the kettlebells are just below the pelvis, the legs slightly bent, the knees almost stationary, and the back always in the neutral position.

KETTLEBELL EXERCISES

- **C |** Extend the hips explosively and, exploiting their momentum, throw the kettlebells up ahead of you. Without drawing the arms away from the trunk, gather the kettlebells to your chest into the rack position.

- **D |** Bend the legs rapidly with a brief, fast, and powerful movement.

(continued)

TRAINING WITH KETTLEBELLS FOR STRENGTH AND MOBILITY

Long-Cycle Clean and Press *(continued)*

- **E |** Extend the legs and, exploiting their thrust, raise the arms above the head. You are in the lockout position. Lower the kettlebells back into the rack position and start from point B. Complete the required repetitions.

Discussion

This is one of the three competition exercises in kettlebell training (though, in competition, the second part of the movement is a jerk and not a push press) and absolutely one of the best for the upper body. It is actually a true total-body exercise: It engages the hip extensor chain, the trapezius, deltoids, triceps, parascapular and paravertebral muscles, and the core. The length of the kinematic chain involved is confirmed also by the effects on the cardiovascular and cardiorespiratory systems, which are driven hard by this exercise (and so trained properly), and also by the rise in basal metabolism after the exercise. The activation mode from low (lower body) to high (upper body) and the downswing that follows make it a fantastic exercise for women with circulation problems (cellulite above all). For the same reason, we also recommend including it in slimming programs for both sexes given that with the same execution we obtain a workout that follows the peripheral heart action (PHA) training method. The long cycle, finally, is one of the best exercises for training stamina and endurance in round-based combat sports or any that takes place over a medium- to long time period. Circle in red, and respect!

KETTLEBELL PUSH-UP

Starting position

- **A |** Adopt the push-up position with the hands on two kettlebells and straighten the body like a plank. The feet are on the ground, the arms straight, the hands grip the kettlebells, and the shoulders are perpendicular to the hands.

Execution

- **B |** Bend the arms and lower your body between the kettlebells with a controlled movement. Keep the body perfectly straight, and then slowly return to the starting position. Complete the required repetitions.

Discussion

This exercise requires control, coordination, balance, and strength. The body must go down as low as possible, attempting to fully stretch the pectoralis, clavicular fascia, and deltoid muscles. The relatively narrow support base of the two kettlebells requires a degree of precision and control we don't find in ordinary push-ups. It is a good exercise to add to the basics or the floor press. It is ideal for sports in which the scapulohumeral joint is subjected to leverage, stretching, and contraction phases, such as wrestling and combat arts.

TRAINING WITH KETTLEBELLS FOR STRENGTH AND MOBILITY

BOTTOM-UP PRESS

Starting position

- **A |** Stand and grip a kettlebell with the right hand.
  Wind up the hip and swing the kettlebell level with the right shoulder, in the bottom-up position, with the handle pointing down and the soma, the sphere, facing up.

KETTLEBELL EXERCISES

Execution

- **B |** Holding the kettlebell tightly in the bottom-up position, raise the arm up, executing a press.
  Slowly lower the kettlebell, keeping the same position.
  Complete the required repetitions.
  Repeat with the other arm.

B

Discussion

Strength in the upper arms starts from the hand grip—I mentioned this in the first part of the book. Just think how many sports require a strong, marked grip: judo, wrestling, combat and martial arts, weightlifting, basketball, baseball, rugby, American football, and boxing. It is the ideal exercise to train the hand-forearm block, a small but fundamentally important kinematic chain. This chain includes all the muscles of the thenar and hypothenar eminence, the flexors and extensors of the fingers, the radial, brachioradial muscle, and all the other flexors and extensors of the forearm.

KETTLEBELL SHRUG

Starting position

- **A |** Stand with your legs slightly bent. Grip a kettlebell with the left hand and bring it into the lockout position; the right arm is abducted laterally, the thumb pointing up.

Discussion

I owe the discovery of this exercise to master Pavel Tsatsouline. In my opinion it is one of the best for strengthening the entire parascapular and paravertebral musculature and for working on posture. The combination of respiration and contraction is most interesting; the exercise does not allow just the muscles mentioned above to work. It also and chiefly allows the activation of the diaphragm, the respiratory muscle *par excellence*, and of the scalene muscles, all at the same time. This is a highly

KETTLEBELL EXERCISES

Execution

- **B |** Inhaling, raise both arms up. Exhaling, return to the starting position. Complete the required number of repetitions, and then switch arms and perform the exercise again on the other side.

B

important factor when talking posture: We will never manage to compensate for postural defects with work on the humerus retractor muscles, for example, if we don't remove all diaphragmatic retractions first. Full respiration, both upper and lower, is the best and most natural exercise for activating the diaphragm in both its upper and lower domes. A word of advice: Don't perform more than 5 repetitions per side, at least at first, followed by a brief pause. Hyperventilation during the workout could lead to pressure loss and dizziness.

KETTLEBELL WALK

Starting position

- **A |** Stand and hold a kettlebell with your right hand and bring it into the lockout position.

Execution

- **B |** Holding the lockout position, contract the abdominal fascia slightly and start walking.
Execute the exercise for the length of time required.

KETTLEBELL EXERCISES

- **C |** Repeat, raising the left arm.

C

Discussion

Simplicity yields the best results. The kettlebell walk is an excellent exercise for posture and for reinforcing the parascapular and paravertebral musculature (especially the humerus retractor and the extrarotator cuff muscles), both activated by the long lever generated by the overhead arm. At the same time, the abdominal fascia is activated to stabilize the torso. For optimal execution, the progression is important. Time first—reach up to 30-40 sec or more—then add weight.

TRAINING WITH KETTLEBELLS FOR STRENGTH AND MOBILITY

DOUBLE CLEAN SQUAT AND PRESS

Starting position

- A | Stand, holding a kettlebell in each hand. The arms should be in front of the hips.

Start in the same way as in the swing. Imagine a jump with no aerial phase.

- B | Flex the pelvis back and wind up the hips (the kettlebells are just below the pelvis; the legs are slightly bent, the knees almost stationary, and the back always in the neutral position).

  Extend the hips explosively and, exploiting their momentum, swing the kettlebells up ahead of you.

  Without drawing the arms away from the trunk, gather the kettlebells to your chest into the rack position.

- C | Bend the legs and, with controlled movement, sit back into a full squat.
- D | Extend the legs explosively and exploit their propulsion to straighten the arms up, executing a press.

  Bring the kettlebells back to the rack position and repeat again.

Discussion

This is a fantastic general conditioning exercise. It features a winning combination: ballistic wind-up phase; action and function of the hip extensor chain (gluteus, femoral muscle, quadriceps); abdominal fascia stabilization; action and function of the scapulohumeral girdle; and stabilization of the paravertebral musculature. It is hard to find muscles that aren't activated in this excellent exercise. All the systems follow in sequence: the cardiovascular and cardiorespiratory systems first, then the others. What was said for the clean and press exercise holds true absolutely for this exercise. This exercise is excellent for women with circulation problems, for slimming programs, and for strength programs (with variable loads, according to the objectives set).

PART III – OBJECTIVES, METHODS, AND TRAINING PROGRAMS

CHAPTER 11

11.1 THE FUNCTIONAL CHOICE

Your body as the best-fitting outfit; a new feeling of efficiency; and technical gestures once unthinkable now become easily-mastered exercises. If you have fully understood the concept of functional training, then maybe you are already feeling all this and experiencing it firsthand. You are only taking your first steps, yet you feel that something is changing, and more will change. I am now forced to dampen your enthusiasm, however, and remind you that functional training is a choice but not an excuse to throw away all you previously practiced in gyms. Actually, its first application is a return to basic exercises, suitably improved and adapted.

Action + Function = Functional training

We must not forget the importance of basic gym exercises such as squats, lunges, pulls, and presses. In this respect, and according to the definition I gave, the performance of weightlifting athletes in clean and jerk and snatch exercises is extremely functional. We have, in fact, an extremely powerful action of the hip extensor chain: a motor action first, then a stabilizing action by the abdominal fascia, and finally, these forces are conducted to the upper body. What do a boxer, a baseball player, a tennis player, and a golfer have in common? Apparently nothing, but if you observe the movement biomechanics, you will find the same concepts previously expressed: wind-up and activation of the hip extensor chain; motor and stabilizing action of the abdominal fascia; and transduction of these forces to the upper body. Have I made myself clear?

The following programs presented in chapters 11 through 13 include bonus exercises which use the following weights: kettlebells, medicine balls, and sandbags. Mastering the exercises in chapter 10 should give you a good foundation for basic form so that if you wish, you can complete the exercises in these programs using various weights. For more details on performing the exercises, see the other volumes in The Ultimate Functional Training Series: *Training With Bodyweight*, *Training With Medicine Balls*, and *Training With Sandbags*.

11.2 STRENGTH TRAINING

We can define strength as the ability to defeat a resistance or to oppose it with a muscular effort (Zatziorskj).

Strength is a conditional ability, which depends about 80% on nerve factors. These factors imply:

- Maximum capacity for recruitment of type II white fibers (IIx especially).
- Maximum development of the central nervous system which, we may remember, takes place approximately by the age of 14.
- The ability to deactivate Renshaw's cells, the cells that act as breakers of the motor message.

The remaining 20% consists of organic and metabolic factors.

- The percentage of type IIa and type IIx white fibers.
- The density, hence the quantity, of white fibers within the transverse section area of the muscle.
- Increase in the diameter of white fibers.
- Improvements in recruitment (see chapter 5).

11.3 STRENGTH-TRAINING PROGRAMS

There are specific programs for strength training. The limit of the programs that follow is that they lack maximal tests and the work on the load percentages for those who pursue such objectives. I have therefore based mine on load progression and on increasing volume and workload by progressively higher-weight percentages within a "wave" program. The positive fact is that they work for everyone.

PROGRAM 1	
WORKOUT A	**WORKOUT B**
Run 10 min	Run 10 min
Squat 3 x 10.8.6 One-leg kettlebell deadlift 3 x 10 + 10	At-the-shoulder lunge with sandbag 3 x 10 + 10 Overhead squat with kettlebell 3 x 10 + 10
Deadlift 3 x 10.8.6 Pull-up 3 x max	Rower with two sandbags 3 x 10 Clean and press with two kettlebells 3 x 15
Horizontal bench press 3 x 10.8.6 Sandbag clean and press 3 x 15	Front shoulder press with barbell 3 x 10 Snatch with kettlebell 3 x 10
Run 10 min	Run 10 min

Training code
Total-body on major areas
Frequency: 2-3 times per week
Duration: 8-9 weeks
Note to workout A: Rotate the pairs of exercises every week so as to distribute the energies equally on all major areas.
Workout A progression: Every two weeks add a set of 6 to the first exercise in each group with a pyramidal method, up to a maximum of 5
Workout B progression: Every two weeks add 1 set to the first exercise in each listed pair.

TRAINING WITH KETTLEBELLS FOR STRENGTH AND MOBILITY

PROGRAM 2	
WORKOUT A	**WORKOUT B**
Run 10 min	Run 10 min
Deadlift 4 x 8.6.6.4 Front squat 3 x 10.8.10	One-leg deadlift 3 x 10 One-leg squat 3 x 10
Horizontal bench press 4 x 8.6.6.4 Pull and press with sandbag 3 x 10	Clean and press with sandbag 3 x 20 Sandbag floor pull 3 x 20
Pull-up 4 x max Push press with two kettlebells 3 x 10	Push press with barbell 3 x 10 Tight grip bench 3 x 10
Run 10 min	Run 10 min

Training code
Total-body on major areas
Duration: 8 weeks
Frequency: 3 workouts per week
Notes to sheet A: Rotate the exercise pairs.

PROGRAM 3	
WORKOUT A	**WORKOUT B**
Run 10 min	Run 10 min
Horizontal bench press 5 x 5; recovery 4 min Low pulley 3 x 10; recovery 2 min	Dumbbell press on fitness ball 3 x 10; recovery 1 min 30 sec Clean and press with kettlebell 3 x 10
Squat 5 x 5 Leg curl on fitness ball 3 x 10	Pull-up 3 x max One-leg deadlift with two kettlebells 3 x 10, each side
Deadlift 5 x 5 Lat machine anterior 3 x 10	Barbell curl 3 x 10 Parallel dips 3 x max
Run 10 min	Run 10 min

Training code
Total-body
Duration: 8 weeks
Frequency: 3 times per week

STRENGTH

PROGRAM 4	
WORKOUT A	**WORKOUT B**
Run 10 min	Run 10 min
Squat 3 x 7-9; 3 x 4-6; 3 x 11; recovery 4 min	Deadlift 3 x 7-9; 3 x 4-6; 3 x 11
Swing with kettlebell 3 x 20	Floor pull 3 x 20
Military press 3 x 7-9	One-leg deadlift 3 x 7-9
Clean with kettlebell 3 x 20	Walking lunge with rotation 3 x 10, each side
Narrow-grip bench press 3 x 7-9	Barbell curl 3 x 7-9
Run 10 min	Run 10 min

WORKOUT C
Run 10 min
Horizontal bench press 3 x 7-9; 3 x 5-7; 3 x 11
Floor press 3 x 20
Clean and press with kettlebell 3 x 7-9
Med ball side lunge with rotation 3 x 10, each side
Snatch with kettlebell 3 x 20, each side
Run 10 min

PROGRAM 5	
WORKOUT A	**WORKOUT B**
Run 10 min	Run 10 min
Power swing with kettlebell 3 x 10 sec	Kneeling jump 3 x 5
Squat 3 x 6; 3 x 3; 3 x 11	Deadlift 3 x 6; 3 x 3; 3 x 9
Pull-up 3 x max	Clean and press with kettlebell 3 x 5-7
Push press with kettlebell 4 x 5-7	One-leg deadlift 3 x 5-7
Barbell curl 3 x 10	Crossover push-up 3 x 10
Run 10 min	Run 10 min

WORKOUT C
Run 10 min
Plyo push-up 3 x 5
Horizontal bench press 3 x 5; 3 x 3; 3 x 9
Low pulley 3 x 10
Leopard plank 3 x 20
Parallel dips 3 x max
Run 10 min

CHAPTER 12

12.1 HYPERTROPHY TRAINING

One whole book on this subject wouldn't be enough. There are one thousand and one studies on hypertrophy, but also no certainties as to the mechanism and the cause/effect of the hypertrophic stimulus. Just think about muscular fibers: They can be white, red, intermediate, totipotent, or satellite; each of these responds to one or more different stimuli. Not to mention the other components of the skeletal muscle: the sarcoplasmic, connective or lipid components, or that huge mystery that the brain still is today, with the cerebellum and nervous system, from which everything departs and where everything ends up. This gray area explains the profusion of techniques and methods, ranging from the scientific to the picturesque or the fanciful. Do we have to make do with what is available? Shall we continue with the approximations and anecdotal fantasies of odd guys in gyms? No, we shan't. We must understand our body, a perfect machine to which no computer, even the most advanced, can be remotely compared. Our body has always adapted according to the function for which it was created and has evolved in the course of millennia.

TRAINING WITH KETTLEBELLS FOR STRENGTH AND MOBILITY

Let's see the priorities then:

1. Training the function of an articular system or a kinematic chain. Do you remember? The purpose, the reason for which that system or chain was built and created and has evolved to the present day.
2. Training the planes involved in the gestures and actions which relate to these systems and kinematic chains. What is the sense of training thighs and glutes with exercises on the frontal plane only (squats and deadlifts) if the hip extensor chain and the coxofemoral joint both share movement ranges on the sagittal and intermediate planes too?
3. Multijoint exercises: There are no monoarticular gestures in daily life.
4. Management and alternation of the loads (i.e., periodization) and the stress induced by them.

This is where I want to start from. I want to integrate an ordinary gym exercise program and its progression with exercises and modifications typical of functional training.

12.2 COSMETIC AND FUNCTIONAL HYPERTROPHY

As I mention in my book *Kettlebell* (Elika Publishers), a dispute is raging in the gym world, a feud which has developed as physical culture has shifted gradually from a performance sport—working on strength and its adaptations—to a sport with purely aesthetic features. The dispute is between cosmetic and functional hypertrophy. Cosmetic hypertrophy, as defined by American athletic coaches, is an increase in muscle mass for its own sake, with the objective of climbing on-stage or exhibiting a well-defined, muscular physique, with no performance purposes. Functional hypertrophy instead is an increase in muscle mass for performance purposes, meaning that it is combined with features such as strength, agility, power, and speed. Where does the main difference between these two cultural extremes lie? In workouts and their adaptations. In workouts we must combine classic basic exercises with functional exercises in order to stimulate different kinematic chains and different motor qualities and skills. As for adaptations, they are connected with functional hypertrophy and involve the central nervous system to a greater degree.

12.3 FUNCTIONAL HYPERTROPHY-TRAINING PROGRAMS

PROGRAM 1	
WORKOUT A	**WORKOUT B**
Run 8 min	Run 8 min
*Horizontal bench press 3 x 10; recovery 2 min Push-up 3 x max; recovery 1 min 30 sec	*Horizontal bench dumbbell press 3 x 10 Leopard push-up 3 x 10
*Front lat machine (without knee pad) 3 x 10 Floor pull 3 x 10	*Rower with sandbag 3 x 10-15 Lacerta push-up 3 x 10
Barbell push press 3 x 10-12	*Squat jump 3 x 5 Walking lunge & rotation 3 x 5 each side
*Front squat 3 x 10 Walking lunge 3 x 10, each side	Frontal stabilizers on forearms 3 x 10 sec Reverse crunch with sandbag 3 x 10
Straight-arm front stabilizers 3 x 10 sec Oblique crunches 3 x 10, each side	Run 8 min
Run 8 min	

Training code
Total-body
Duration: 6-8 weeks
Progression: every week add 1 set to the exercises marked by *

HYPERTROPHY

PROGRAM 2	
WORKOUT A	**WORKOUT B**
Run 8 min	Run 8 min
Horizontal bench press 3 x 10.8.6; recovery 2 min Leopard push-up 3x10, each side; recovery 1 min 30 sec	*Push-up on kettlebells 3 x max Barbell push on fitness ball 3 x 10
Lat machine middle grip (without knee pad) 3 x 10.8.6 Rower with two sandbags 3 x 10, each side	*Sandbag floor pull 3 x 10 Rower with two kettlebells 3 x 10 Sandbag clean and press 3 x 10
*Clean and press with two kettlebells 3 x 10 Diagonal press with med ball 3 x 10, each side	*Squat and press with kettlebell 3 x 10 One-leg kettlebell deadlift 3 x 10, each side
*Front squat with barbell 3 x 10 Walking lunge with rotation 3 x 10, each side	Side plank with rotation 5 x 10, each side
Run 8 min	Run 8 min

Training code
Total-body
Duration: 6-8 weeks
Progression: every 2 weeks add 1 set to the exercises marked by * (add 1 set of 6 reps to the exercises with pyramidal method)

PROGRAM 3	
WORKOUT A	**WORKOUT B**
Run 8 min	Pull-up 3 x max
*Front squat 3 x 5 At-the-shoulder lunge with sandbag 3 x 10, each side Power swing 3 x 10	*Reverse row: horizontal tractions from the multipower bar 3 x max Lacerta push-up 3 x 20
Plyo push-up 3 x 5-7 *Horizontal bench press 3 x 5 Push-up 3 x 10	*Double jerk with two kettlebells 3 x 5-7 Diagonal press with med ball 3 x 10, each side Bent press 3 x 7, each side
Barbell curls from the preacher position (kneeling on a mat, the pelvis off the heels) 3 x 7-9	Parallel dips 3 x max Leopard plank 3 x 30 sec Reverse rope crunch 3 x 10
Sandbag reverse crunch 3 x 10 Side plank 3 x 10 sec, each side	Run 8 min
Run 8 min	

Training code
Split routine
Duration: 6-8 weeks
Progression: every 2 weeks add 1 set to the exercises marked by *

TRAINING WITH KETTLEBELLS FOR STRENGTH AND MOBILITY

PROGRAM 4	
WORKOUT A	**WORKOUT B**
Rope skipping 5 min	Run 10 min
Walking lunge with barbell 3 x 5, each side	Bent press with kettlebell 3 x 7, each side
Front squat and press 3 x 7-9	Pull-up 3 x max
Burpee 3 x 20	Sandbag floor pull 3 x 10
Dumbbell push 3 x 5	Clean and jerk with two kettlebells 3 x 7
Leopard push-up 3 x 20	Push press with kettlebell 3 x 15
Narrow-grip bench press 3 x 5	Barbell curl 3 x 5-7
Reverse rope crunch 3 x 20	Leopard plank 3 x 30 sec
Side plank with rotation 3 x 10, each side	Side plank with twist 3 x 10, each side
Rope skipping 5 min	Run 10 min

Training code
Split routine
Duration: 6-8 weeks
Progression: every week add 1 set to the first exercise for each muscle group, up to a maximum of 5 sets

CHAPTER 13

13.1 SLIMMING TRAINING

Those who follow me know that slimming is a metabolic condition with several "parents". There are many organic lipolytic paths, meaning there are different methods to start losing body fat. First of all let's clarify what we mean by slimming. We don't simply mean a decrease in weight. Scales are of little use in *slimming* (greatly overweight subjects excepted), because they don't measure the real decrease in body-fat percentage.

How to define slimming then? *Slimming* is a decrease in the lipid organic fractions, especially the subcutaneous and visceral ones. Let me start with a commonplace observation we should, however, keep in mind: There is no slimming without a suitable eating regimen, or at least it is extremely difficult. This point may appear obvious, but it happens to be the basic reason for a lack of results. Having said this, let me be clear that circuit work is suitable for other types of adaptations, too, from hypertrophy to strength. The neurogenic and muscular components involved are determined by the type of training stimulus.

13.2 LIPOLYTIC PATHS

Here is a brief review of the training stimuli to be "administered" (that term isn't chosen at random) to activate different lipolytic paths:

1. **Muscle tone training**

Muscle tone is a very low-intensity electrical message that is always present in any active muscle, even at rest. This is typically a nerve adaptation, which can be reached by classic strength training. Strength training increases muscle tone over time; this generates an increase in the subject's basal metabolism and an increase in the oxidative work on body fats when at rest, too.

2. **Training for hypertrophy**

Many people ask me what hypertrophy and slimming have in common. When completing an exercise to exhaustion, lactate production indicates a hormonal response by

- the growth hormone: proteolytic and lipolytic response;
- catecholamines: adrenaline and noradrenalin (lipolytic response); and
- thyroid hormones: lipolytic response.

But is this enough? There is actually more to this; for example, we know that by doing interval work up to the lactate threshold, we influence EPOC heavily. All this translates in a metabolic increase which lasts for several hours after training (depending on the intensity of the exercise, up to 12, 16, even 24 hours and more) with a 10-15% increase in body-fat burning at rest!

3. **Aerobic training**

The oxidative paths in Krebs cycle are essential in providing the amount of oxygen necessary for lipolysis. Low-intensity aerobic work is indispensable for obese or greatly overweight subjects in the initial phase of training. It is important for beginners, too, though over time the intensity will have to increase progressively, reaching interval training and circuits. Regarding circuits, cardio-fit training, peripheral heart action, and circuit training methods are particularly beneficial.

Further progressions of these are:

- Blitz circuits, for their ability to put all organic systems under heavy stress in a very short time, reaching oxygen debt immediately.
- Timed circuits, for the efficient management of the gesture or gestures being performed.

13.3 CIRCUIT TRAINING

I have been talking about circuit training as the training for the future for at least a decade. You can stimulate highly differentiated systems and organic structures with one single method. Circuit training is essential for general physical preparation for any performance sports-specific training, for strength and hypertrophy training, and for creating a slimming strategy for everyone. The method variations make this a highly diverse type of training, never boring and with a level of intensity ranging from beginners to athletes. The best-known methods are circuit training, cardio-fit training, PHA training, Blitz circuits, timed circuits, and boot camp. Let's take a look at them.

13.3.1 Circuit training

Organized by the US Army around 1956, circuit training consists of a sequence of exercises, varying from 6 to 10 or more, to be repeated with little or no rest between each of them. The execution of one entire sequence of exercises is called a circuit. At the end of each circuit, you can choose between passive or active recovery before starting again.

The number of circuit runs varies from 2 to 10.

PROGRAM 1	PROGRAM 2
TOTAL-BODY PROGRAM FOR EVERYONE	FOR BEGINNER WOMEN
Run 10 min	Run 10 min
Push-up 1 x 10	Swing with kettlebell 1 x 20
Crunch 1 x 10	Push-up 1 x 5-10
Clean with sandbag 1 x 10	Walking lunge 1 x 5, 10, each side
Arms plank 1 x 10 min	Arms plank 1 x 10 sec
Walking lunge 1 x 10	Squat and press with kettlebell 1 x 5/10
Reverse rope crunch 1 x 10	Clean and press with sandbag 1 x 10
Recovery 2 min	Walk 2 min
Repeat the sequence 5 times	Repeat the sequence 3-5 times
Run 10 min	Run 10 sec

SLIMMING

PROGRAM 3	PROGRAM 4
FOR BEGINNER MEN	FOR BEGINNER MEN
Run 10 min	Run 10 min
Push-up 1 x 10	Leopard plank 1 x 10
Rope crunch 1 x 10	Plyo push-up 1 x 5
Floor pull 1 x 10	Reverse rope crunch 1 x 10
Forearm plank 1 x 10 sec	Clean and press with kettlebell 1 x 10
Front squat 1 x 10	Side plank with twist 1 x 10, each side
Reverse rope crunch 1 x 10	Squat and press with kettlebell 1 x 10
Rower with sandbag 1 x 10	Swing 1 x 20
Leopard plank 1 x 10 sec	Recovery 2 min
Recovery 2 min	Repeat the sequence 5 times
Repeat the sequence 5 times	Run 10 min
Run 10 min	

PROGRAM 5	PROGRAM 6
DYNAMIC EXERCISES FOR BEGINNER WOMEN	DYNAMIC EXERCISES FOR BEGINNER MEN
Run 10 min	Run 10 min
Jumping jack 1 x 10	Skip 1 x 10 min
Skip 1 x 10 sec	Push-up 1 x 10
Swing 1 x 10	Jumping jack 1 x 10
Squat and press 1 x 10	Clean and press with sandbag 1 x 10
Rope crunch 1 x 10	Burpee 1 x 10
Push press with kettlebell 1 x 10	Squat and press with kettlebell 1 x 10
Sandbag reverse crunch 1 x 10	Sandbag reverse crunch 1 x 10
Clean and press with sandbag 1 x 10	Recovery 2 min
Recovery 2 min	Repeat the sequence 3-5 times
Repeat the sequence 3-5 times	Run 10 min
Run 10 min	

PROGRAM 7	PROGRAM 8
FOR INTERMEDIATE MEN	FOR INTERMEDIATE WOMEN
Swing 1 x 20	Run 10 min
Leopard push-up 1 x 20	Swing 1 x 20
Side plank with twist 1 x 10, each side	At-the-shoulder walking lunge with sandbag 1 x 10, each side
Burpee 1 x 20	Clean and press with kettlebell 1 x 10
Pull and press with sandbag 1 x 20	Swing 1 x 20
At-the-shoulder walking lunge with sandbag 1 x 10, each side	Burpee 1 x 20
Side plank 1 x 10 sec, each side	Floor pull 1 x 20
Recovery 2 min	Reverse rope crunch 1 x 20
Repeat the sequence 5 times	Push press 1 x 10
Run 10 min	Recovery 2 min
	Repeat the sequence 3-5 times
	Run 10 min

PROGRAM 9	PROGRAM 10
FOR ADVANCED MEN	FOR ADVANCED WOMEN
Swing 7 min (alternate one-armed and two-armed)	Swing 7 min
Burpee 1 x 20	Burpee 1 x 20
Push-up with two kettlebells 1 x 20	Leopard plank 1 x 20
Med ball side lunge with rotation 1 x 10, each side	Push-up 1 x max
Leopard plank 1 x 20	At-the-shoulder lunge with rotation 1 x 10, each side
Pull-up 1 x 20	Side plank with rotation 1 x 5, each side
Squat and press with kettlebell 1 x 10-20	Clean and press with kettlebell 1 x 10-20
Rower with sandbag 1 x 20	Squat and press with kettlebell 1 x 10
Side plank with rotation 1 x 5, each side	Reverse rope crunch 1 x 20
Recovery 2 min	Rower with sandbag 1 x 20
Repeat the sequence 5 times	Recovery 2 min
Swing 7 min	Repeat the sequence 3-5 times
	Swing 7 min

13.3.2 Cardio-fit training

Cardio-fit training is a circuit training method that alternates aerobic phases—on cardio machines or with aerobic exercises (running, rope skipping, walking)—and anaerobic phases. Initially, the cardio phase is used as active recovery after an exercise phase. The circuit's level of difficulty is increased gradually, heightening the intensity of both the anaerobic and the aerobic phases. Cardio-fit training is a typical interval training method. This is its main strength.

In 1998 it was the subject of a study carried out by Neri, Paoli, and Velussi, who compared its slimming effects to those of the classic method of aerobic training. In the course of the study, they selected two groups of athletes, both composed of beginners. The first group trained on cardio machines only, while the second group performed cardio-fit training with triceps and abs exercises only. The plicometer test results were rather surprising: the degree of slimming in both groups was similar but on triceps and abs the cardio-fit group slimmed down twice as much! At a time when the diatribe on localized slimming was at its peak, the study had a lot of recognition and was the basis for a series of further studies which confirmed its results.

TRAINING WITH KETTLEBELLS FOR STRENGTH AND MOBILITY

PROGRAM 1	PROGRAM 2
FOR BEGINNER WOMEN	FOR BEGINNER MEN
Cardio 10 min	Cardio 10 min
Squat 1 x 5 Lateral clean (quadrupedal) 1 x 10, each side Repeat 2 times without stopping	Push-up 1 x 10 Rope crunch 1 x 10 Repeat 2-3 times without stopping
Cardio 5 min	Cardio 5 min
Step-up 1 x 5, each side Backward clean (quadrupedal) 1 x 10, each side Repeat 2 times without stopping	Squat 1 x 5-7 Straight-arm stabilization 1 x 10 sec Repeat 2-3 times without stopping
Cardio 5 min	Cardio 5 min
Press with med ball 1 x 10 Straight-arm stabilization 1 x 10 sec Repeat 3 times without stopping	Press with sandbag 1 x 10 Rope diagonal crunch 1 x 5, each side Repeat 2-3 times without stopping
Cardio 5 min	Cardio 5 min
Rower with sandbag 1 x 10 Rope crunch 1 x 10 Repeat 3 times without stopping	Floor pull 1 x 10 Forearm stabilization 1 x 10 sec Repeat 2-3 times without stopping
Cardio 10 min	Cardio 10 min

SLIMMING

PROGRAM 3	PROGRAM 4
FOR INTERMEDIATE WOMEN	FOR INTERMEDIATE MEN
Cardio 10 min	Cardio 10 min
Squat jump 1 x 5 Reverse rope crunch 1 x 10 Repeat 3 times without stopping	Med ball crossover push-up 1 x 6, each side Reverse rope crunch 1 x 10 Repeat 3 times without stopping
Cardio 5 min	Cardio 5 min
One-leg kettlebell deadlift 1 x 5, each side Box squat 1 x 5 Repeat 3 times without stopping	Clean and press with sandbag 1 x 10 Side plank with twist 1 x 10, each side Repeat 3 times without stopping
Cardio 5 min	Cardio 5 min
Floor pull 1 x 10 Side plank with twist 1 x 5, each side Repeat 3 times without stopping	Walking lunge 1 x 10, each side Side plank with rotation 1 x 5, each side Repeat 3 times without stopping
Cardio 5 min	Cardio 5 min
Med ball diagonal press 1 x 10, each side Reverse rope crunch 1 x 10 Repeat 3 times without stopping	Rower with two sandbags 1 x 10 Rope diagonal crunch 1 x 10, each side Repeat 3 times without stopping
Cardio 10 min	Cardio 10 min

PROGRAM 5	
FOR ADVANCED WOMEN	
Run 10 min	Cardio 5 min
Kettlebell overhead walking lunge 1 x 10, each side Lateral clean (quadrupedal) 1 x 10, each side Repeat 3 times without stopping	Clean and press with sandbag 1 x 10 Push-up 1 x 10 Repeat 3 times without stopping
Cardio 5 min	Cardio 5 min
Lu.Be.Lu.Be. 1 x 2 rounds, alternating Kettlebell swing 1 x 20 Repeat 3 times without stopping	Floor pull 1 x 15 Side plank with rotation 1 x 5, each side Repeat 3 times without stopping
	Cardio 10 min

TRAINING WITH KETTLEBELLS FOR STRENGTH AND MOBILITY

PROGRAM 6	
FOR ADVANCED MEN	
Run 10 min	Cardio 5 min
Burpee 1 x 10 Leopard crunch 1 x 10, each side Repeat 4 times without stopping	Clean and press with two kettlebells 1 x 10 Squat and press with two kettlebells 1 x 10 Repeat 4 times without stopping
Cardio 5 min	Run 10 min
Sandbag floor pull 1 x 20 Plyo push-up 1 x 7 Repeat 4 times without stopping	

PROGRAM 7	PROGRAM 8
GENERAL PHYSICAL PREPARATION FOR WOMEN	GENERAL PHYSICAL PREPARATION FOR MEN
Run 10 min	Run 10 min
Swing 1 x 20 Squat and press with two kettlebells 1 x 10 Repeat 4 times without stopping	Leopard push-up 1 x 20 Sandbag floor pull 1 x 20 Repeat 4 times without stopping
Cardio 5 min	Cardio 3 min
Clean and press with sandbag 1 x 15 Rower with sandbag 1 x 15 Repeat 4 times without stopping	Med ball half-kneeling position with rotation 1 x 10, each side Side plank with rotation 1 x 10, each side Repeat 4 times without stopping
Cardio 5 min	Cardio 3 min
Push-up 1 x 10 Side plank with rotation 1 x 7, each side Repeat 4 times without stopping	Kettlebell squat and press 1 x 10 One-leg kettlebell deadlift 1 x 10, each side Repeat 4 times without stopping
Cardio 5 min	Cardio 3 min
Burpee 1 x 10 Rope V-crunch 1 x 10, each side Repeat 4 times without stopping	Rower with sandbag 1 x 20 Kettlebell renegade row 1 x 10, each side Repeat 4 times without stopping
Run 10 min	Run 10 min

13.3.3 Peripheral heart action (PHA) training

Created as a bodybuilding technique by Bob Gajda, PHA training has been subsequently applied to circuit training, as a method within the method. It can be applied to all the circuit training programs we have seen so far. It consists of an alternation of selected exercises, working on muscular areas distant from one another.

The distance between the areas stimulates the cardiorespiratory and cardiovascular systems strongly, increasing their activity. Their job is to provide oxygen and metabolites (which are then removed) to the muscles during the exercise. The lipolytic effect is decidedly greater.

Here are some examples of PHA training.

PROGRAM 1	PROGRAM 2
FOR BEGINNER WOMEN	FOR BEGINNER WOMEN
Cardio 10 min	Cardio 10 min
Squat 1 x 10 Med ball press 1 x 10 Repeat 3 times without stopping	Swing 1 x 20 Squat and press 1 x 10 Repeat 3 times without stopping
Cardio 5 min	Cardio 5 min
Walking lunge 1 x 5, each side Floor pull 1 x 10 Repeat 3 times without stopping	At-the-shoulder walking lunge with sandbag 1 x 10, each side Push-up 1 x 10 Repeat 3 times without stopping
Cardio 5 min	Cardio 5 min
Push-up with knee support 1 x 5 Rope V-crunch 1 x 5, each side Repeat 3 times without stopping	Kettlebell push press 1 x 10 One-leg kettlebell deadlift 1 x 10, each side Repeat 3 times without stopping
Cardio 5 min	Cardio 5 min
Kettlebell swing 1 x 10 Straight-arm plank 1 x 10 sec Repeat 3 times without stopping	Rower with sandbag 1 x 15 Reverse rope crunch 1 x 10 Repeat 3 times without stopping
Cardio 10 min	Cardio 10 min

TRAINING WITH KETTLEBELLS FOR STRENGTH AND MOBILITY

PROGRAM 3	PROGRAM 4
FOR BEGINNER MEN	FOR BEGINNER MEN
Cardio 10 min	Cardio 10 min
Squat 1 x 10 Push-up 1 x 10 Repeat 3 times without stopping	At-the-shoulder sandbag squat 1 x 10, each side Med ball crossover push-up 1 x 7, each side Repeat 3 times without stopping
Cardio 5 min	Cardio 5 min
Floor pull 1 x 10 One-leg kettlebell deadlift 1 x 10, each side Repeat 3 times without stopping	Sandbag floor pull 1 x 20 At-the-shoulder sandbag lunge 1 x 10, each side Repeat 3 times without stopping
Cardio 5 min	Cardio 5 min
Med ball diagonal press 1 x 10, each side Plank 1 x 10 sec Repeat 3 times without stopping	Rower with two sandbags 1 x 20 Reverse rope crunch 1 x 15 Repeat 3 times without stopping
Cardio 5 min	Cardio 5 min
Burpee 1 x 5 Rope crunch 1 x 10 Repeat 3 times without stopping	One-leg kettlebell deadlift 1 x 10 Forearm plank 1 x 20 sec Repeat 3 times without stopping
Cardio 10 min	Cardio 10 min

PROGRAM 5	
FOR INTERMEDIATE WOMEN	
Run 10 min	Cardio 5 min
Burpee 1 x 10 Leopard plank 1 x 10, each side Repeat 3 times without stopping	Swing 1 x 30 Reverse rope crunch 1 x 20 Repeat 3 times without stopping
Cardio 5 min	Cardio 5 min
At-the-shoulder sandbag lunge 1 x 10, each side Push-up 1 x 10 Repeat 3 times without stopping	Sandbag floor pull 1 x 20 Med ball diagonal press 1 x 10, each side Repeat 3 times without stopping
	Cardio 10

SLIMMING

PROGRAM 6
FOR INTERMEDIATE MEN

Run 10 men Swing 1 x 30 Double jerk 1 x 15 Repeat 3 times without stopping Cardio 5 min Kettlebell squat and press 1 x 20 Med ball crossover push-up 1 x 10, each side Repeat 3 times without stopping	Cardio 5 min Sandbag floor pull 1 x 20 Burpee 1 x 20 Repeat 3 times without stopping Cardio 5 min Side plank with twist 1 x 10, each side Kneeling jump 1 x 10 Repeat 3 times without stopping Run 10 min

PROGRAM 7	PROGRAM 8
FOR ADVANCED WOMEN	FOR ADVANCED MEN
Run 10 min Squat and press 1 x 10 Leopard plank 1 x 10, each side Repeat 3 times without stopping Run 5 min Lunge jump 1 x 7, each side Clean and press with sandbag 1 x 20 Repeat 3 times without stopping Run 5 min Squat jump 1 x 5 Plyo push-up 1 x 5 Repeat 3 times without stopping Run 5 min Med ball diagonal press 1 x 10, each side Reverse rope crunch 1 x 15 Repeat 3 times without stopping Run 10 min	Run 10 min Kettlebell squat and press 1 x 20 Leopard plank 1 x 20 Repeat 3 times without stopping Run 5 min Burpee 1 x 20 Leopard push-up 1 x 20 Repeat 3 times without stopping Run 5 min Kneeling jump 1 x 10 Side plank with rotation 1 x 10, each side Repeat 3 times without stopping Run 5 min Sandbag floor pull 1 x 20 Plyo push-up 1 x 10 Repeat 3 times without stopping Run 10 min

13.3.4 Blitz circuits

Widespread test evidence suggests we should bear in mind the following factors as the keys to reaching different objectives.

SLIMMING

1. Gradual work on EPOC is essential; increases in EPOC are related to the intensity of the exercise rather than its duration.
2. Increase in metabolic "horse power" through an increase in lean mass; the lean mass increase is chiefly promoted by lactacid work.
3. Muscle tone work; muscle tone increase (a much underestimated concept) is connected to alactacid training.
4. Lipolytic hormones activation (GH, testosterone, catecholamines, thyroid hormones) through lactacid–alactacid work.

TONING

1. Lean mass increase.
2. Muscle tone increase.
3. Anabolic hormones activation (GH, IGF-1, IGF-2, testosterone, FGF, insulin) through lactacid–alactacid work.
4. Training should concentrate exclusively on alactacid–lactacid workouts.

Starting from these premises I have developed blitz training circuits that are fast, intense, and effective. They last up to 30 min, and this is more than enough! Blitz circuit effectiveness is related to its intensity; basic exercise selection will be key, as well as the loads, which will point in the direction of the desired objective (slimming, toning, muscle tone, or hypertrophy).

SLIMMING

PROGRAM 1	PROGRAM 2
SLIMMING	**SLIMMING FOR WOMEN**
Cardio 5 min: ideally walking, (stationary) steps, running, horizontal bike	Cardio 5 min: ideally walking, (stationary) steps, running, horizontal bike
Dynamic deadlift 1 x 15 Rower with barbell 1 x 15 Front squat 1 x 15 Front shoulder press 1 x 15 Repeat 3-5 times without stopping	Front squat 1 x 10 Rower with barbell 1 x 15 Walking lunge 1 x 5, each side Front shoulder press 1 x 15 Repeat 3-5 times without stopping
Cardio 5 min	Cardio 10 min
Note: The barbell must be the same light weight for all the exercises in the circuit. The subject will pick up the barbell at the start of the blitz and will not set it down until the end of the workout.	**Note:** The execution should not be too quick. It is important to find your own cadence and rhythm and to maintain it, improving gradually.

PROGRAM 3	PROGRAM 4
TONING	**ATHLETIC TRAINING**
Cardio 5 min: ideally walking, (stationary) steps, running, horizontal bike	Running or rope skipping 5 min
Squat 1 x 10 Front shoulder press 1 x 10 Walking lunge 1 x 10, each side Bar tractions (dips) 1 x 10 Repeat 5 times without stopping	Power swing (very heavy load) 1 x 10 Horizontal bench press 1 x 5 Power swing 1 x 10 Squat 1 x 5 Power swing 1 x 10 Chin-ups 1 x 5-7 Repeat 3-5 times without stopping
Cardio 5 min	Cardio 5 min
Note: Once you have grasped the blitz concept, it is important to move beyond these outlines and adapt them to our clients. Blitz circuits are extremely versatile and can be adapted to any subject, even beginners, by fine-tuning loads and intensity.	

TRAINING WITH KETTLEBELLS FOR STRENGTH AND MOBILITY

PROGRAM 5	PROGRAM 6
FOR FEMALE SUBJECT WITH CELLULITE OR OTHER CIRCULATORY PROBLEMS	FOR MMA
Cardio 8 min Swing 1 x 10 Push-up 1 x 10 Front squat 1 x 5 Rower with sandbag 1 x 10 Step-up (two steps) 1 x 5, each side Repeat 3-5 times without stopping Cardio 8 min **Note:** The swing must be executed fast but with a rather light load. Load the front squat with 8 RM. The step-up exercise is essential to work on plantar arch circulation and help the venous blood flow.	Rope skipping 8 min Kettlebell clean and press 1 x 15 Burpee 1 x 10 Kettlebell squat and press 1 x 15 Bar pull-up 1 x max Med ball lunge with rotation 1 x 10, each side Push-up 1 x 15 Repeat 5-10 times without stopping Rope skipping 8 min **Note:** Plan a mini-recovery at the end of each circuit. Question: How long does a MMA bout last for? You will have to continue working non-stop on the circuit for the same amount of time. From here on, managing your energy levels throughout the bout will not be a problem.

PROGRAM 7	PROGRAM 8
GENERAL PHYSICAL PREPARATION	GENERAL PHYSICAL PREPARATION FOR WOMEN
Cardio 10 min Kettlebell squat and press 1 x 15 Sandbag snatch 1 x 10 Med ball diagonal press 1 x 10, each side Crossover lunge 1 x 10, each side Rower with sandbag 1 x 20 Side plank with twist 1 x 10, each side Repeat 5-10 times without stopping Cardio 10 min	Cardio 10 min Kettlebell power swing 1 x 10 At-the-shoulder sandbag squat 1 x 10, each side Floor pull 1 x 20 One-leg kettlebell deadlift 1 x 10, each side Push-up 1 x 10 Repeat 5-10 times without stopping Cardio 10 min

SLIMMING

13.3.5 Timed circuits

The timed circuit concept was inspired by kettlebell work. In this type of circuit training you don't count sets and reps but only work for the preset time. You can apply this methodology, fine-tuning the exercises and the repetitions, on any type of subject: sedentary, intermediate, advanced, or athletes. You can also manage intensity (i.e., the effort expended in each single set), exercise by exercise, according to the student's degree of fitness and his or her special needs. Since the objective is long-duration work, managing the right level of intensity is clearly of utmost importance. For this reason I suggest starting with a load of about 10 RM, with only 5-6 reps per set.

PROGRAM 1	
ANTI-CELLULITE	
Uphill walking 15 min (3% slope; 2.8-3.1 mi/h [4.5-5 km/h]) Coreboard step-up 1 x 5, each leg Quadruped backward leg lift 1 x 10, each leg	Leg curl with fitness ball 1 x 5 Swing with kettlebell 1 x 10 Repeat for 10-20 min without stopping Uphill walking 15 min (3% slope; 2.5 mi/h [4 km/h])

Note: If the subject is a beginner, you will start with a 5-min workout, gradually increasing the time with each workout. Execution throughout the circuits will have to be extremely careful to maximize the training stimulus. The versatility of timed circuits and circuit training in general makes for virtually infinite combinations.

PROGRAM 2	
MULTI-DISTRICT WOMAN	
Uphill walking 10 min (3% slope; 2.8-3.1 mi/h [4.5-5 km/h]) Kettlebell or dumbbell swing 1 x 15 Quadruped backward leg lift 1 x 10, each leg Step-up on two steps 1 x 5, each leg Straight-leg quadruped lateral lunges 1 x 5, each leg Repeat for 10 min without stopping Cardio 5 min or active recovery 3 min Plank stabilization 1 x 20 sec Oblique crunches 1 x 5, each side	Lateral stabilization 1 x 15 sec, each side Reverse crunch 1 x 5 Repeat for 10 min without stopping Cardio 5 min Push press with dumbbells 1 x 6 Renegade row 1 x 5, each side Push-up 1 x 6 Floor pull 1 x 6 Repeat for 10 min without stopping Walking 10 min (cool-down)

TRAINING WITH KETTLEBELLS FOR STRENGTH AND MOBILITY

PROGRAM 3	
TOTAL BODY	
Walking 10 min (warm-up)	Frontal stabilization 1 x 20 sec
Front squat 1 x 5	Repeat for 10 min without stopping
Floor pull 1 x 6	Cardio 5 min
Walking lunge 1 x 5, each leg	Kettlebell clean and press 1 x 6
Push press with kettlebell 1 x 6	Oblique rope crunches 1 x 10, each side
Repeat for 10 min without stopping	Swing with kettlebell 1 x 15
Cardio 5 min	Reverse rope crunch 1 x 10
Sandbag pull and press 1 x 6	Repeat for 10 min without stopping
Push-up 1 x 6	Walking (cool-down) 10 min
Rower with sandbag 1 x 6	

Note: Timed circuit training for advanced subjects marks the evolution from sportsperson to athlete; it forces you to refine your technique—your energy management and economy of gestures on the one hand and reduction of risks and increase in benefits on the other.

PROGRAM 4	
FOR THE INTERMEDIATE ATHLETE	
Run 10 min	At-the-shoulder sandbag lunge 1 x 6
Horizontal bench press 1 x 6	Med ball burpee 1 x 6
Front squat 1 x 6	Repeat for 10 min without stopping
Low pulley 1 x 6	Active recovery 3 min
One-leg kettlebell deadlift 1 x 5, each side	Kettlebell swing 1 x 10
Repeat for 10 min without stopping	Plyo push-up 1 x 5
Active recovery 3 min or cardio 5 min	Kettlebell deadlift 1 x 6
Kettlebell push press 1 x 6	Sandbag floor pull 1 x 6
Rower with sandbag 1 x 6	Repeat for 10 min without stopping
	Cardio 10 min

13.3.6 Boot camps

Boot camp training is a circuit training method based on the military courses used by soldiers worldwide for their operational training. It reached Italy, riding the popularity wave of training methods such as cross-fit and kettlebell training. It is an excellent, engaging group workout system. Boot camp training features a great variety in terms of exercise setting, exercise equipment, training intensity, and the management of groups ranging in numbers from 10 people to several hundreds. Boot camp training relies on the coach's ability in setting the course, planning the sequence and duration of exercises, and on the enthusiasm of fitness lovers ready to work out anywhere, whether in a park or a garage. I will never forget my experience at the summer 2012 boot camp in San Diego, California for the IDEA World Convention.

Warm-up: a 4 km (2.5 mi) run to the USS Midway aircraft carrier, moored in San Diego harbor. One hour of intense body-weight exercises led by Todd Durkin and his staff, then another 4-km cool-down run back to the San Diego Convention Center. Coming back to us, how can you set up a functional boot camp in a gym? This is actually rather simple. A lot depends on the number of people involved and the method used.

We shall therefore distinguish different approaches, based on a different number of stations according to how many the participants are. There are essentially three variables in this kind of circuit training:

1. the exercises
2. the exercise execution time
3. the recovery time between each station

The **exercises** must be extremely simple, especially for beginners and in each boot camp's initial circuits.

Execution time varies with each exercise. What does it depend on? On the objectives of the people you are training. Are you dealing with a group of athletes practicing lactacid or mixed sports (with energy delivery lasting from 30 sec and up)? Workout time will be 30-40 sec per station (as training progresses, you may increase this).

Are you dealing with a group of athletes practicing alactacid sports (power, expressions of strength, and explosiveness for 5-20 sec) ? Plan stations of 10-20 sec, up to a maximum of 30 sec. What about beginners, fitness lovers, and subjects with no competitive yearnings? Start with simple exercises lasting a maximum of 20 sec.

TRAINING WITH KETTLEBELLS FOR STRENGTH AND MOBILITY

Moving from one station to another will be the circuit's active recovery time. This will have to be carefully measured out according to the subjects you are training. With athletes, the time can be progressively shortened, from 20 sec or less. You can actually turn the transfer from one station to another into an exercise; for example, you can reach the next station in a walking lunge, leopard plank, or leopard push-up. With beginners or occasional gym patrons, recovery time should definitely be higher. If the workout time at the station is, for example, 20 sec, recovery time between stations should be at least 30 sec. The last factor is space. The limit of an indoor boot camp is the space available. This is why I will restrict my indications to the number of people statistically more likely, given the usual size of gyms.

2 BOOT CAMP STATIONS
Groups between 8 and 20 people

Split the people into two distinct groups: Group 1 and Group 2. Group 1 (G1) will do a standing body-weight workout. Group 2 (G2) will work on mats. Assign an exercise to both groups. Execution time: Begin with 20 sec per station. Warm-up time: 10 min.

Circuit 1	Circuit 3
G1: squat 1 x 20 sec G2: crunch 1 x 20 sec Switch the exercises and repeat. Repeat this pair of exercises three times per group, with a 20-sec recovery time between exercises.	G1: floor pull 1 x 20 sec G2: reverse crunch 1 x 20 sec Switch the exercises and repeat. Repeat this pair of exercises three times per group, with a 20-sec recovery time between exercises.
Circuit 2	Circuit 4
G1: Walking lunge 1 x 20 sec G2: arm stabilization 1 x 20 sec Switch the exercises and repeat. Repeat this pair of exercises three times per group, with a 20-sec recovery time between exercises.	G1: leopard push-up G2: forearm stabilization 1 x 20 sec Switch the exercises and repeat. Repeat this pair of exercises three times per group, with a 20-sec recovery time between exercises.

SLIMMING

4 BOOT CAMP STATIONS
Groups between 16 and 40 people

Split the participants into four groups:
G1, G2, G3, G4.
Set up four exercise stations: A, B, C, D.

Assign a muscle area to each station:

A = dynamic legs
B = core training
C = classic legs
D = trunk and upper body

Develop four exercises per station.

A
- Jumping jack
- Skip
- Starter
- Burpee

B
- Crunch
- Straight-arm plank
- Reverse crunch
- Plank with twist

C
- Squat
- Walking lunge
- Crab
- Lunge with rotation

D
- Push-up
- Lacerta push-up
- Leopard push-up
- Floor pull

Rules
1. Assign one group per station.
2. Assign and demonstrate to each group the first exercise in each station (Jumping jack, crunch, squat, push-up).
3. Start the clock: 20 sec to execute the maximum number of reps.
4. After 20 sec, stop the exercise and signal the station change.
5. Each group has 20 sec to transfer to the next exercise station.
6. Start the clock again for another 20 sec.
7. Repeat the sequence so that each group will complete the four stations circuit (Jumping jack, crunch, squat, push-up) three times.
8. Now pause so that athletes can recover and drink some water; then show each group the second exercise in each station (skip, straight-arm plank, walking lunge, lacerta push-up)
9. Start the cycle again, completing four circuits, with three sets per exercise.

ETHICS AND CONCLUSIONS

If you have come this far, then probably you are in it up to your neck… like me. Functional training improves your mind and body, makes you more open and observant, and, makes you a better person (why not?).

Your body will become a perfectly tailored outfit, your mind always lucid, and your senses focused to the max. You will enjoy your training and every moment of your life with an intensity you have never experienced before.

If you have come this far, please read these last few lines.

ETHICS OF THE FUNCTIONAL ATHLETE

1. Train by using your body.
2. Keep your eyes open, watch and discover new exercises.
3. Always keep your mind open.
4. Continue along your course: Improvement has no limits.
5. Compare your method, you will find certainties.
6. Love who you are and what you do.

Happy training, everybody!

CREDITS

Cover design: Kristina Ehrhardt, Anja Elsen

Cover photos: © Guido Bruscia and Thinkstock/iStock

Photos: Chapter images on p. 18, 19 32, 33, 35, 44, 45, 64, 80, 91, 111: Shutterstock (www.shutterstock.com)
Chapter graphics: © Thinkstock/iStock

The rights to all photos remain with the publisher.

Layout: Kristina Ehrhardt, Anja Elsen

Typesetting: www.satzstudio-hilger.de

Copyediting: Elizabeth Evans